US AND THEM
The Psychology of Ethnonationalism

Report No. 123

US AND THEM
The Psychology of Ethnonationalism

Formulated by the
Committee on International Relations

Group for the Advancement of Psychiatry

BRUNNER/MAZEL *Publishers* • New York

Library of Congress Cataloging-in-Publication Data

Us and Them.

(Report; no. 123)
Bibliography: p. 129
Includes index.
1. Ethnicity. 2. Nationalism—Psychological aspects.
3. Identity (Psychology) I. Group for the Advancement
of Psychiatry. Committee on International Relations.
II. Series: Report (Group for the Advancement of Psychiatry: 1984);
no. 123. [DNLM: 1. Ethnopsychology. W1 RE209BR
no. 123 / GN 270 U84]
RC321.G7 no. 123 [GN495.6] 616.86 s [305.8] 87–17872
ISBN 0–87630–481–1
ISBN 0–87630–480–3 (soft)

Published by
BRUNNER/MAZEL, INC.
19 Union Square West
New York, New York 10003

MANUFACTURED IN THE UNITED STATES OF AMERICA

10   9   8   7   6   5   4   3   2   1

STATEMENT OF PURPOSE

THE GROUP FOR THE ADVANCEMENT OF PSYCHIATRY has a membership of approximately 300 psychiatrists, most of whom are organized in the form of a number of working committees. These committees direct their efforts toward the study of various aspects of psychiatry and the application of this knowledge to the fields of mental health and human relations.

Collaboration with specialists in other disciplines has been and is one of GAP's working principles. Since the formation of GAP in 1946, its members have worked closely with such other specialists as anthropologists, biologists, economists, statisticians, educators, lawyers, nurses, psychologists, sociologists, social workers, and experts in mass communication, philosophy, and semantics. GAP envisages a continuing program of work according to the following aims:

1. To collect and appraise significant data in the fields of psychiatry, mental health, and human relations;
2. To reevaluate old concepts and to develop and test new ones;
3. To apply the knowledge thus obtained for the promotion of mental health and good human relations.

GAP is an independent group, and its reports represent the composite findings and opinions of its members only, guided by its many consultants.

US AND THEM: THE PSYCHOLOGY OF ETHNONATIONALISM was formulated by the Committee on International Relations. The members of this committee are listed on page vii. The members of the other GAP committees, as well as additional membership categories and current and past officers of GAP, are listed on pp. 141–147.

ACKNOWLEDGMENTS

The Committee on International Relations gratefully acknowledges its indebtedness to members, fellows, guests, and consultants who assisted us in formulating this Report.

The study could not have been undertaken without the help of consultants from other fields. In the early stages of our work, we were ably guided by Gerald L. Gold, Ph.D., Department of Anthropology, York University, Downsview, Ontario, and Daisy M. Tagliacozzo, Ph.D., Professor of Sociology, University of Massachusetts.

In 1980 the Committee was fortunate to have enlisted the help of Howard Stein, Ph.D., and anthropologist and teacher in the Department of Family Medicine at the University of Oklahoma Health Sciences Center and editor of the Journal of Psychoanalytic Anthropology, who worked with us through the completion of the Report in 1986. His studies of Slovak- and Ruthene-Americans in western Pennsylvania and America's White Ethnic movement of the late 1960s and early 1970s, interests that widen into "Pan-isms" around the world, attracted our Committee's attention. Moreover, our work was greatly complemented by his concern with psychogeography, the psychological uses of ethnicity, and the unconscious aspects of organizational and cultural group dynamics, especially in how group symbols and practices come about and are maintained.

Mohamed Shaalan, M.D., Professor and Chairman of the Department of Neurology and Psychiatry, Al-Azhar University, Cairo, Egypt, was a special guest of the Committee and added valuable perspectives on our subject matter. Former members of our Committee who returned to visit us and contributed generously are David N. Ratnavale, M.D., Bryant Wedge, M.D., and Louis C. English, M.D. Other guests were psychiatrists Otto Kernberg, M.D., and

Thomas Valk, M.D., who contributed helpful commentary in the final stages of preparation for the Report.

As is the custom in the preparation of GAP reports, numerous members of the organization reviewed our draft and made invaluable contributions and corrections. Any errors that remain are our own.

In 1978 the Committee began its study of ethnonationalism under the chairmanship of Ronald Wintrob, M.D., who transferred to another Committee of GAP in 1980. From then until completion of the Report in 1986 the Committee was chaired by Francis F. Barnes, M.D.

The Committee is grateful to Mrs. Virginia Kennan and Mrs. Alberta Zimmisch for their editorial assistance.

> No man is an Illand, intire of it selfe; every man is a peece of the Continent, a part of the maine; if a Clod bee washed away by the Sea, Europe is the lesse, as well as if a Promontorie were, as well as if a Mannor of thy friends or of thine owne were; any mans death diminishes me, because I am involved in Mankinde; And therefore never send to know for whom the bell tolls; It tolls for thee.

> JOHN DONNE

CONTENTS

US AND THEM
The Psychology of Ethnonationalism

1

INTRODUCTION

Being one with the community confers great benefits, ranging from personal sustenance and even survival to participation in magnificent cultural achievement. But paradoxically, group-belonging can also lead to killing and to the destruction of culture in war. War has always been a critical issue for the survival of man as an individual, as a family, and as nations of peoples, but now it has also become an issue for man as a species.

The biopsychosocial forces that underlie group-belonging are crystalized in our times as ethnonationalism. If man dies as a species, it is because as an ethnonationalist he is too much one with his community and too divided from other communities. Such is the healing and harming bivalency of ethnonationalism that if we regard it as a cancer, then we must remember that cells prior to becoming cancerous were not bad. They are good cells gone awry; patriotism can become ethnonationalism.

Man in the heat of battle may have little doubt about why he is at war. But in more tranquil moments man the philosopher has long wondered why. In our century, Einstein, seeing the rapidly growing technological ability of man to make ever-more destructive war, asked Freud (1933/1964): Why? In asking the question he claimed that he himself was "free of national feelings" and suggested a simple structural solution: renunciation of national sovereignty in favor of international institutions. He thought the psychological barriers to such a course lay not only in the vested interests of political and industrial leaders (the minority of the population), but also in the majority. "Because man has within him a lust for hatred and destruction" (p. 201).

Freud agreed. He pointed out that man, like the entire animal kingdom, always solved conflicts by force, muscular force, tools, and even "better" weapons. To control such a force would require the superior strength of a unified community—which conceivably could come about as a result of war—a latter day "precious Pax Romana." He considered that the force of ideals or ideology (he instanced the Communist ideology) cannot today replace actual force. He then turned to a discussion of Eros, the life instinct, and its complex relationship to the destructive instinct. He, of course, favored all measures that would help intellect and culture triumph over the cruelties and aesthetic humiliations of war.

What is most interesting to note in Freud's views on this matter is an emphasis on biology. "We are pacifists because we are obliged to be for organic reasons" (p. 214). He appears to have anticipated some of the concepts of modern sociobiology studies when he commented: "The process is perhaps comparable to the domestication of certain species of animals, and it is undoubtedly accompanied by physical alterations; but we are still unfamiliar with the notion that the evolution of civilization is an organic process of this kind" (p. 214). He saw culture as strengthening the intellect over the instincts and noted the need for an elite group of independent thinkers to lead the masses.

Since Freud's time other behavioral science disciplines have been dealing with the subject of human divisiveness at their own levels of observation and analysis. We note, however, that there has been little contribution to the field from psychoanalytic psychology. From a number of standpoints this is surprising. This discipline has not been shy in examining such fields as social movements, art, the personalities of leaders, history, and so on. It is curious that psychoanalysis, which concerns itself with the deepest examination of man's relationship to others in the microcosms of personal life, the family, and more recently in small group relations, has paid so little attention to the larger ethnonational context of human relations, the context in which wars occur.

Cultural psychiatry has shown great interest in the different expressions of psychiatric syndromes and their epidemiology in various cultures and ethnic groups. Although the field has long been concerned with such fundamental and influential subjects as child rearing and education, it has been slow to concern itself with the metapsychological essence of cultural differences and divisiveness.

The International Relations Committee of GAP became interested in the nature and development of man's sense of his ethnicity and nationalism as an outgrowth of our study of man's disposition to make war (GAP, 1978). We found that war participants explained their behavior not only from the standpoint of preserving their lives and lands, but also as deriving from a sense of obligation and belonging to their ethnic and national groups. The latter motivation was sometimes sufficient in itself, that is, even in the absence of any direct threat to life and property. The powerful psychological components of ethnonationalism beg for understanding.

Our historical and clinical case studies of individuals for whom ethnicity is intensely experienced suggest a series of psychological perspectives on the relationship, in essence the continuity, between the individual and the group. We see a continuity that has its origins in long-forgotten biological union with and dependence on mother for physical survival and physiological homeostasis. The continuity draws upon later developmental stages of gradual differentiation from mother. During these stages there is a gradual growth of a facultative capacity to affiliate and dissociate. This faculty is not the product of any single time or age-limited developmental stage but is built upon series of developmental stages. The process of individuation is constantly subject to fluctuation along a normal progression/regression axis and forms a prototype for an adult life affiliation/separation function in interpersonal and intergroup relations.

The ability of the human to achieve self-development and independence while retaining his proclivity to merge, whether regressively or as a progressive assimilative social phenomenon, appears to have important underpinnings in biological development. We note that in the case of certain species, especially marine species, the individuals are so continuous with one another it is difficult to determine which is the unit of the species, the individual, or the colony.

The philosopher in everyone wonders, as he sees his offspring born and develop: "Am I so unique? Am I just a link in the large human chain that goes on generation after generation?" We suppose that musings of this kind are universal and represent conscious correlates of the survival thrust of the species. And if our philosopher uses more sophisticated terms he may wonder: "Am I a cell of the larger animal? Is the real individual the gene, Weismann's germ plasm, passed on from the germ cell in which an individual originates in direct continuity to the germ cells of succeeding generations?"

Feelings of and belief in intergenerational continuity find spiritual expression in such simple animistic ideas as the migration of souls. They may also find expression in more sophisticated religious teachings, as, for example, the traditional Christian idea that the church comprises the living and the dead, the Community of Saints.

We have formed the impression that the sense of ethnicity also rests on sets and fragments of mental representations relating to the ego ideal and the negative ego ideal (roughly, what a person should and should not be) acquired during the earliest stages of the child's enculturation. Though at first it is the parents' bodily and emotional qualities the infant learns, he soon incorporates along with these, the ideas and ideals with which his parents shape him. These first educators (for such they are, whether or not they think of themselves so) make free use of their own ethnic history, heroes, and so forth. This ensures that significant numbers of children in any community will grow up with at least some common denominator of ethnic identity and attachment, which will assure the preservation of that community's particular cultural coloration. This is an area in which some of the elusive links between individual and group psychologies may be found.

Though psychiatrists have been conducting small groups and making useful observations for many years, we must confess that group theory lags. The step from understanding individual behavior to understanding group behavior is difficult and fraught with traps. Since Freud's venerable speculations on group psychology, the field has taken some modest strides including the delineation by Bion (1961) of certain "basic assumptions" that are shared by small groups. Our thesis is in essential agreement with, and attempts to extend, his observation that the individual and the group perform functions for each other that replicate the early life functions of child and parents.

In Bion's "dependency group" the individual's sense of weakness and inadequacy reactivates the tendency—so clearly observable in early life—to idealize the leader or parent as omnipotent and to extract, from him or her, power and perfection. Members of the group are drawn together by their shared sense of weakness and their demand upon one another—and upon the leader especially—for help against an unfriendly outside world. We see, and attempt in later chapters to illustrate, the same processes at work in larger ethnic and national groups.

The "fight-flight" process Bion described in small groups is probably also basic to the larger group and repeats some of the dynamics of the early mother-child relationship, especially as the child comes to deal with the existence of others beyond the mother-child dyad. We refer of course to the "stranger reactions" infants display in two prominent stages, at about three months old and again at eight months. Although these reactions, which appear to be subjectively dysphoric, diminish and change with time, there remains in all of us through childhood and into adult life this innate tendency to feel comfortable with the familiar person and uncomfortable with the stranger. This facilitates identification with the familiar and hostility to the outsider. Denial of in-group hostility and its externalization and projection onto the outsider play into the hands of ethnonationalism's divisiveness.

In the third of Bion's group dynamic principles, the "pairing assumption," the group beneficently expects two of its members to pair off and reproduce to assure the survival of the group. The relevance of this dynamic process to the perpetuation of ethnic and national groups is biological and obvious. Israel's preoccupation with its youth and their future role as saviours and continuers of the nation is simply one of the better known but universal instances of this psychology.

Basic in our thesis is the idea that individual and group are one and continuous. The individual may feel and act independently much of the time, but in large degree his behavior is not only a component of the group behavior, but is also to a great extent determined by the group, often even a direct expression of the group. This is certainly the lesson in so much of our current study of the family, where analysis of child behavior often reveals it to be a direct or compromise enactment of a drive or impulse of one or both parents who have not been able to acknowledge or manage such impulses successfully themselves. Even in normal family processes much of the behavior of the offspring is determined by the particular coloration of the family structure.

Every family has a kind of gestalt of itself, its history, and concepts of its place in society, of class, religion, occupations, ideas, and so on. To the extent that these values are held by many or all other families in a society, they become a common denominator of ethnicity to which all members of the group can respond as if to the family itself. Families that are exceptional and in a minority in some respect such as religion may still feel a deep commitment to the other social values that they share with their neighbors. The values to which we refer usually involve ego ideals and negative ego ideals, aspirations, and images of historical figures and events, which constitute shared mental representations. The communalization of introjects encourages the sharing of the same psychology of the continuity of self and other, whether lover, family, or group. These widely held sets of mental representations are then available for evocation by skillful leaders through the manipulation of allusions, symbols, rituals, and so on.

The intuitive and charismatic ability of certain individuals to key into a community's shared values and immediate concerns is fundamental in the emergence of leaders. The ability of such a leader to manipulate and even create new sets of psychological images or introjects assures a continuing dynamic between leader and nation that has the ability to change both leader and nation.

The psychological forces that determine the development of ethnic and national identity in the human personality interact powerfully with numerous social forces and structures. For example, language, religion, cultural symbols, and myths may be regarded as transmitters and amplifiers of ethnonational affiliation and distinctiveness (Mack, 1983). They are repositories of those elements by which the group defines itself and by which the individual at least in part defines himself. Reciprocal feedback loops and reinforcement between individual and group are evident in all the attendant phenomena.

These transmitters and amplifiers are powerful tools for establishing boundaries, that is, accomplishing the inclusiveness and exclusiveness of each group. They are capable of extraordinary refinement in fulfillment of their function, which often entails establishing what Freud (1930/1961) referred to as the "narcissism of minor differences." This is a particularly important and even desperate exercise when the competing peoples are very similar in a number of respects and occupy the same or contiguous territories. It can be carried to such ludicrous extremes that the participants must surely be wise to themselves, as, for example, Protestant and Catholic farmers in Northern Ireland each saying of the other that "he digs with the wrong foot."

In this Report we can look only briefly at some of the transmitters and amplifiers of ethnonationalism; there is an abundant literature on each and all of them, though perhaps not quite in this context.

Race and associated biological theories. The line of descent probably owes its preeminent position as a determinant of inclusiveness to the centrality of the family. Even when the scale becomes large, the literal and metaphorical connection to the family is not forgotten, as in "the family of English speaking nations." Differences in color and anatomy inflate the virulence of racism by dehumanization and, in Erikson's language, lead to pseudospeciation. Less than human qualities are ascribed to "inferior" races, and whole theories of history have been elaborated based on invidious comparisons between one's own race and those of others.

Language. From early infancy language is both a unifier and divider of people. The sounds mother and infant make to each other may rival sight and touch as modulators in the intricate process of development. Much that is unique in the cooing and baby talk of a mother and infant duet is of necessity, over the course of time, lost in favor of the language of the community. But even so, the principle of specialness is not lost; for millenia, it has been possible for people to identify as strangers, on the basis of accent or idiom, those who may live only a few miles away, and so to include, exclude, persecute, and so forth. Even the powerful influences of radio, television, and travel have not quite homogenized language.

Religion. When viewed as a system of shared beliefs and controls on behavior, religion can be seen to originate in the family and serves as a bridge to join the individual and the family to society. Because of the universality and truth of some spiritual experiences such as love and peace, religion can connect all peoples and transcend ethnonationalist divisions. But all too often religion, especially as an institution, is subject to manipulation by the times and human leaders. It becomes an instrument for reducing personal and group tension by including all good within and externalizing all bad.

Cultural symbols. Cultural symbols such as those related to foods, flags, and songs, are powerful amplifiers in the formation of a nationalistic identity. On the one hand, an ethical respect for the richness and diversity of other cultures can be used to connect peoples one to another. On the other hand, symbols such as the swastika, hammer and sickle, crescent, cross, and Star of David can also be used to mobilize exclusiveness and hatred.

Psychogeography. Psychogeography consists of the use of natural and man-made social space as symbols of the self and of others (Niederland, 1956, 1957, 1971; Stein, 1984b, 1985; Volkan, 1979). Rivers, lakes, mountains, islands, highways or streets, walls, and railroad tracks are but a few of the markers of group-boundaries by which group members experience themselves and others. These formations help groups crystalize their sense of "who-ness" in terms of a sense of their "where-ness," for example, the difference between the positive feeling from having grown up on the "right" side of the tracks and the negative feeling from having grown up on the "wrong" side of the tracks. The Berlin Wall is a powerful psycho-geographic symbol; for many Americans the Mason-Dixon line likewise remains a powerful psychogeographic symbol.

Cultural space plays out and represents themes in developmental time—hence the need for a *psycho*geographic perspective. Such spatial referents can be experienced as lying along a range from highly abstract and metaphorical to literal and concrete. Size, shape, expansion, contraction, and the permanence of one's territory all perform symbolic functions; human territorialism thus cannot be reduced to a concern for physical survival apart from psychic survival. People often come to associate their security and fate with the vicissitudes, strength, or vulnerability of these boundaries that separate "us" and "them."

Myth and history. Alouph Harevan, a sociologist of ethnonationalism, once said that in descriptions of nationalism the truth of history is the first victim. Each group elaborates kernels of past happenings (the factual aspect may be minimal) and embroiders tales of the heroism of one's own group and of the perfidy of others. In comparison with one's own group, others are mean, cowardly, and generally lacking in human virtue. Aggrandizing versions of the history of one's group are provided by parents, teachers, and national leaders and through the mass media. We have commented on the uncanny capacity of some leaders to play on primitive, developmental, differentiating psychic representations to mobilize the members of a nation against other peoples. It is a great challenge to psychiatrists, as it is to historians and statesmen, to sort out the real pain, bloodshed, and hurt that are the result of nationalistic wars from the psychic projection and leader-inspired collective manipulations that play on the perceptions of history.

Ideology. Ideologies are broad, generally vague, value-laden schemata that leaders of nations, drawing on theorists who appeal to their political persuasions, use to structure and simplify collective human realities. Visionary ideologies can connect peoples and transcend nationalistic differences if they are truly inclusive, but generally the ethical-political-economic pseudotheory that comprises a particular ideology is used in a narrow, nationalistic fashion to pursue the "interests" or purposes of a particular national group, especially as defined by its leaders. An overarching ideology and restructuring of reality are often implicit in what appear superficially to be practical programmatic moves, realpolitik, or humanitarian policies. Ideologies operate profoundly in both East and West in current dangerous confrontation. Ideologies are powerful mobilizers of the deep individual and group psychological forces that bind personal identities to collective purposes. It is a particular responsibility of the humanist to find ways to increase awareness of the polarizing nature of ideologies, to shed light on situations in which groups are unaware of how they are being manipulated by divisive leaders who play on their emotions through false visions and through the creation of terror-laden spectres of dehumanized enemies.

Technology. Technology is, by itself, idea-less and ethically and psychologically neutral. It is ever more apparent that the communications media have become powerful tools with which to influence people, including inflaming ethnonationalist differentiation or, we may hope, bringing groups together.

Of great concern to us is the amplifying effect technology has on the irrational in man. Within everyone, no matter how rational, there persists in some degree traces of the magical thinking of early childhood. The infant is tormented by feelings of weakness, unimportance, and frustrated rage when mother is absent too long. At her return—and his gratification—he experiences feelings of merging with her and possessing her enormous power or magic. Such omnipotent thinking and feeling will in the course of growth be modified by experience and reason. But these feelings persist and are manifested in such arenas as supernatural beliefs and science fiction where Superman and Buck Rogers are well-established exemplars. Modern technology has accomplished such miracles not only for Buck Rogers but for all of us, so that it seems to offer man the prospect of omnipotence and the conquest of his deepest fears.

Such expectations appear to be fueled by, for example, the death-defying technological "miracles" of modern medicine. So, too, weapons technology may stir within us unwarranted hopes for omnipotence in battle. As we remind ourselves that our health cannot be perfect and youth everlasting, we must also recognize that the scenario of our invincibility in a Star War exists only in what we may call the madness of technology—not in reality.

New weapons of mass destruction make obsolete the conventional means by which ethnonational groups have defended their singularity and survived. Our species cannot assume that the quantum increase in the power of human destructiveness will not evoke or activate irrational belligerency. To date man has shown some caution about his new weapons, but history is not lacking in examples of wars undertaken in the grandiose certainty induced by the discovery of a new weapon. So nuclear weapons and the madness that may be associated with them make the need for greater understanding of ethnonationalism's psychological sources ever more pressing.

A question inevitably arises: To what extent is man conscious of the psychological processes involved in ethnonationalism? We observe that man has constantly changing levels of awareness of the biological and psychological underpinnings of his union with his fellow man. It would appear that the value our society places on individuation in the quest for functional maturity requires and achieves only partial and variable suppression of the individual's consciousness of his feelings of continuity with others. Changing external circumstances readily mobilizes or reduces individual as well as social consciousness of ethnic unity.

The continuity between man and his society calls for a variable balance between independent behavior and merging in group behavior. The faculty to vary these behaviors finds its origin and prototypes in the stages of separation/individuation in early infancy.

Childhood thrusts toward separation and individuation, alternating with periods of rapprochement and conformity with mother's behavior and demands, form a model for later-life ability to act either independently or in concert with others—even to the extent of merging unquestioningly in regressive group behavior such as may occur in the course of war.

Feelings of solidarity and behavior that merges with the group tend to be high in the face of exigent events and low during socially tranquil times. The structure of society is also a significant factor in these phenomena. Communities such as chronically beleagured minorities, nomadic tribes, and economically marginal subsistence farmers appear to be more constantly aware of their group identity with little emphasis on the singularity of the individual. In contrast to our dominant Western society where the human unit is thought to be the individual, society itself is the unit. A practical reflection of these attitudes is found in the differing relative values given to the legal rights of the individual and the rights of society.

The disposition of Western man to experience his humanity singularly (i.e., individually) appears to have its roots in cultural and historical developments that are now firmly established aspects of our culture and cast their mark on our child rearing and education. Among these we identify the Judeo-Christian emphasis on individual moral responsibility for behavior. The associated doctrine of free will and its corollary teaching that a child attains to free will and certain responsibilities and privileges at particular ages, serve to separate the child from the family and so from the community. While it may be fairly argued that this whole process has contributed to the creation of a splendid civilization, it must be conceded that it has also placed on the individual the burden of greater isolation from supportive society as he has repressed his feelings of continuity with that society. The development of monotheism has made man as lonely as God.

The era of the Enlightenment further reinforced the singularity of man at the rational level. The new emphasis on science and reason entailed intellectual effort which, though it could be learned in groups, required solitary exercise. Again it would seem that this important intellectual component of the magnificent edifice of Western civilization was achieved at the cost of man's sacrificing some of his participation in society as he went his individual way.

We now witness crises in our civilization that drive large numbers of individuals and their leaders back from their singular moral and intellectual development into intense feelings of ethnic and national solidarity, where uncontrolled merger processes may result in regressive suspension of moral and intellectual judgment, which stand in great contrast to our cultural traditions and ideals.

Some of ethnonationalism's consequences are so heinous that it is difficult to understand how ordinarily decent people engage in them. We hope in this work to shed more light on this unhappy state by examining the mental processes that underlie the fine, changing, and sometimes absent lines between man and society.

A prodigious descriptive literature on ethnicity and nationalism has accumulated during the past century from various fields, including history, political science, anthropology, and sociology. Developmental and social psychology have offered some insights also. While we appreciate these diverse contributions, we propose in this Report to examine the psychology of ethnicity on an intimate level and from a particular developmental viewpoint to ask: What is ethnicity? How does one develop a sense of his ethnicity? What does it do for and to people? How is it used by individuals, families, groups, and nations? How does this useful affiliative disposition became dangerous?

In attempting to answer these questions, we draw upon psychoanalytic understanding of individual development. The psychological processes to which we refer derive from various, and perhaps all, stages of early life development. These include the earliest need for physical union and physiological homeostasis, symbiosis, the development of inanimate, and later, more mature forms of object relations, and the idealized union of romantic love. The metapsychology involved includes Freudian concepts, the observations and theories of object relations authors such as Mahler and Winnicott, the formulations of the analysts of narcissism, Kohut and Kernberg, together with the ideas of Blos and Erikson on adolescence. We do not see these as competing explanations but rather as being serially or simultaneously active, often complementing or synergistically enhancing one another. However, we have not limited our conceptual framework to the strictly intrapsychic or even interpersonal concepts traditionally associated with psychoanalysis but are especially interested in applying them to the individual's development of ethnicity in family and group processes.

This work does not pretend to be the last word on the psychology of ethnonationalism. Indeed, it does not even attempt to be a comprehensive psychoanalytic statement on the subject. It is simply an effort to apply one mode of understanding man to a problem of mankind. Although we do not try here to integrate our thesis with the findings of other interested disciplines, we nevertheless believe the thesis to be integrative in nature rather than alternative.

In extrapolating from individual to group psychology, we know well that we are on difficult and controversial ground. Even our method (we should perhaps say "way" instead of "method") of extrapolating cannot be called scientific, involving as it does a mix of facts, speculations, and analogies. The relationship between theories of individual and group behavior is so problematical that some experts deny that there is any relationship. Many contend that we must await the development of new tools with which to study the issue. We proceed on the commonsense view that it is difficult to conceive of a psychology of human groups that is unrelated to the psychology of the individual. No doubt further studies will shed light on many basic questions we have not addressed. Are there not processes of group formation that are common to a number of species? What are the implications of animal-herd formation for human-group formation? We must press on even as we await with interest the answers to such questions.

This Report is an attempt at a scholarly yet clinically informed account of a series of universal phenomena. The individual's sense of "I"ness proceeds to "we"ness, which in turn has implications for intergroup and international relations. Our study is not invalidated if, epistemologically, one mode of understanding these phenomena is not the only mode possible.

One may well question the pertinence of ethnic case material drawn from clinical and societal settings. Ethnic material in clinical cases would be innocuous if not altogether gratuitous were it not that people constantly assign ethnic labels to intrapsychic parts and conflicts. Ethnic facts are not merely neutral; they are hotly valued by their proponents and devalued by their opponents.

The reader may conclude that we are on less firm ground in our speculations on the psychology of ethnicity in larger historical groups. Can one really "psychoanalyze" an entire nation? We are at once ambitious in our goal and humble about the extent to which we have attained it; we do not ask the reader to suspend his critical judgment as we build a new conceptual tool to examine international relations—only that he have the patience and good will to follow us stepwise through an admittedly complex and tenuous argument. The reader eager to see the application of object relations theory to international relations early in this Report will be disappointed, for it is only in the final chapters that we examine the psychodynamics of ethnic and national groups and the further relevance of these dynamics for international nuclear confrontation.

Following this introductory chapter we review briefly the conceptualization of ethnicity and nationalism from the viewpoint of the many disciplines that have examined them. After this comes a lengthy theoretical chapter that explains the important concept of object relations, some of its biological substrate, its part in forming the individual's sense of ethnic identity, and its role in group affiliations. It may prove to be a difficult chapter even for those with some background in psychology. We apologize for its complexity and the psychoanalytic jargon which we have tried to keep to a minimum. We trust the general reader will understand that a first presentation of our thesis must pay full tribute to theory. He may wish to go through this chapter lightly and come to understand its message as we discuss its ramifications in subsequent chapters. Following our theoretical presentation, we deal with ethnicity in the individual in a chapter divided in three sections. The first of these reviews contributions from cognitive developmental psychology in building group members' perceptions of themselves and of others. The next section presents clinical vignettes to illustrate the role of ethnicity in shaping individual lives and the manner in which ethnicity is used by people in resolving personal and interpersonal conflict. The third section deals with the role of object relations in the interaction between the leader and the group. A chapter is devoted to historical and current examples of the dynamics of ethnic and national groups and of intergroup relations. In our conclusion we offer some thoughts on the implications of this study for understanding and reducing group conflict.

2

CONCEPTS OF ETHNICITY AND NATIONALISM

Here we examine the psychology of the affiliative processes involved in ethnicity and nationalism, but what we say can be applied to other social groups and processes such as those of race, religion, sex, age, and occupation. We begin by reviewing some of the definitions and concepts of ethnicity and nationalism.

Ethnicity

The term *ethnic* comes from the Greek *ethnos,* which means a company, people, or nation (Webster, 1977). Along with such related terms as *ethnicity* and *ethnocentrism,* the term *ethnic* suggests a gestalt of interrelated primordial bonds, kinship, affinity, attachment, and grounds for self-esteem (Stein, 1979). Many authorities recognize the subjective experience of ethnicity as part of the self-definition of a person and note that each individual has shared perceptions of the distinctiveness of his ethnic group and a sense of common historical experience. There is also continuity through biological descent and the sharing of common social and cultural conditions. Peterson (1980) remarks that even when there is no full conscious-ness of ethnicity, group members are at least latently aware of having common interests. Even when ethnic identification is not expressed, there can be a feeling that the language and traditions shared with one's fellows are unique.

Most writers on this subject recognize external or objective criteria as well as self-defining or subjective ones, but criteria for ethnicity may be applied a little differently in different contexts, even by the same writer. For example, Greeley (1974) writes about

ethnic groups being "non-social class collectivities" like "those created by diversities in religion, race, and national origins" (p. 172).
With McCready (1975), he wrote that an ethnic group is "a large
collectivity based on presumed common origin, which is, at least
on occasion, part of a self-definition of a person, and which also
acts as a bearer of cultural traits" (p. 210). Most definitions of
ethnicity and nationalism combine them. Shibutani and Kwan
(1965) seem to improve on Max Weber's classic definition of an
ethnic group as a human collectivity based on an assumption of
common origin, real or imagined, when they define it as applied to
"those who conceive of themselves as being alike by virtue of
common ancestry, real or fictitious, and who are so regarded by
others" (p. 47).

Objective criteria by which nonmembers define an ethnic group
stress physical characteristics and some degree of cultural and
social commonality (Cohen, 1978). These many factors may include
race, language, surname, marriage, family relations, kinship, religion and philosophy, politics, education, economic status, dress,
cuisine, arts and crafts, volunteer associations, and games (Cohen,
1978; Gittler, 1977). Members of any one group may have only
some of these factors in common.

When people are assigned to groups on both subjective and
objective grounds, ethnicity creates boundaries for inclusiveness
and exclusiveness. Individuals may have overt and distinct behavioral
affiliations such as those announced by the type of dress or the
language used, but it is the societal designation that makes them
members of a certain ethnic group (Gittler, 1977). Ethnicity has no
existence apart from interethnic relations. This is illustrated in
Genet's play *The Blacks*, in which the notion of *black* has no meaning apart from *white* (Genet, 1960).

Anya Peterson Royce (1982) adds a dynamic element:

> Any definition of ethnic group or ethnic identity must be
> composed of both subjective and objective components and
> must also support the notion that ethnic groups are eminently
> mutable, providing yet another reference group with which
> the individuals can vary their social strategies. (p. 33)

We would add that individuals have repertoires of identities that can be drawn on in changing circumstances; and they have affiliative faculties that can alter the objects of attachment as circumstances require. These objects of attachment are not just ethnic groups but include the local community, the nation, and the profession or religion practiced—any grouping that stirs affiliative feelings based on shared identity.

Most individuals have many overlapping sets of loyalties that make for multiple and at times conflicting identities. One's ethnic identity may coexist with awareness of belonging to a given age group, sex, religion, profession, or nation, but identity boundaries separate those to whom one feels a sense of kinship and obligation from those to whom one feels unrelated and who may serve as what Volkan calls "suitable targets of externalization" (Volkan, 1986).

Reminick (1983) suggests that ethnicity can be studied from six perspectives: the standpoint of environment, such as culture, trends of change, and pressures to assimilate; levels of operation, such as the prevailing social structure, the sophistication of symbols, and personality patterns; operative levels, such as those involving physical traits, types of group interaction, the family, the sense of ethnic honor, and art; approved ethnic modification, as in assimilation and adaptation; causes and functions of ethnicity; and functional modes, as in typical reactions to crisis (Reminick, 1983; Stein, 1985).

Over the millennia civilized man has come to value cultural diversity. Harold Isaacs (1975) notes that personal identity is enriched by what Francis Bacon called the "idols of the tribe"—symbolic meanings given to group differences in body, name, language, art, history, religion, and nationality. To be complete, a theory of ethnicity must also be a theory of human groups and a theory of change (Stein, 1985).

Distinctiveness and uniqueness are universally attributed to the ethnically different. George DeVos (1975), an anthropologist, defines the ethnic group as

> a self-perceived group of people who hold in common a set
> of traditions not shared by the others with whom they are
> in contact. Such traditions typically include "folk" religious

beliefs and practices, language, a sense of historical continuity, and a common ancestry or place of origin. The group's actual history often trails off into legend or mythology, which includes some concept of an unbroken biological-genetic generational continuity, sometimes regarded as giving special characteristics to the group. (p. 9)

Likewise, according to Max Weber each ethnic group has "belief in a specific 'honor' of their members, not shared by outsiders, i.e., the sense of ethnic honor" (quoted by Parsons, Shils, Naegele, & Pitts, 1961, p. 307).

According to LeVine and Campbell (1972):

> *Ethnocentrism* is the technical name for this view of things in which one's own group is the center of everything, and all others are scaled and rated with reference to it. Folkways correspond to it to cover both the inner and the outer relation. Each group nourishes its own pride and vanity, boasts itself superior, exalts its own divinities and looks with contempt on outsiders. Each group thinks its own folkways the only right ones, and if it observes that other groups have other folkways, these excite its scorn. Opprobrious epithets are derived from these differences. . . . For our present purpose the most important fact is that ethnocentrism leads a people to exaggerate and intensify everything in their own folkways which is peculiar and which differentiates them from others. It therefore strengthens the 'folkways.' (p. 8)

At the heart of ethnicity is the feeling of *being special*. People create cultural distinctions to keep one group from being confused with another, and group members exaggerate the ways in which they differ from others in order to denigrate the others, setting themselves up as a superior "pseudospecies" (Erickson, 1966). Thus the enemy, who may not only be hated but also destroyed, is made inanimate. Tragically, as groups "discover" themselves to be special and superior to others, they behave as though they are unaware that all groups engage in this kind of assessment—and for the same reason. All draw attention to their culture and direct it away from the vulnerable identity core they use culture to defend. What a paradox—the insistence on uniqueness is universal; only the cultural trimmings differ, and the core—and core purpose—of identity remains the same.

Nationalism

The word *nation* comes from the Latin *nasci* (to be born), and from this stem comes *natio* (birth), which has the transferred meaning of *tribe, race, people*. Distinguishing nationalism from ethnicity, Gittler (1977) notes that ethnic groups are unorganized, being without internal structure although having a system of symbols and values. Nations, on the other hand, possess organization that creates roles, positions, and status. Gittler (1977) allows that most nations contain more than one ethnic group and that nationality has many meanings and connotations. The terms *nationalism* and *nationalist* are usually used in connection with a recognized national entity, but they may appear in connection with members of an ethnic group that aspires to become an independent state as is the case with the Basques, Palestinians, and others.

Boyd C. Shafer, a student of nationalism, offers definitions of it drawn from a variety of sources (Shafer, 1982) and emphasizes consciousness, citing the declaration of Carlton J.S. Haynes that nationalism is "fusion of patriotism with a consciousness of nationality" (p. 23) English scholars of the Royal Insititute of International Affairs define it as a consciousness, on the part of individuals or groups, of membership in a nation, or of a desire to forward the strength, liberty, or prosperity of a nation. Hans Kohn sees nationalism as a state of mind "in which the supreme loyalty of the individual is felt to be due the nation state" (Shafer, 1982, p. 23).

Shafer (1976) notes four structural and objective "beliefs and conditions" characterizing nationalism and six that are purely psychological. The former include the possession of or desire for a certain territory; cultural commonality in language, customs, manners, and literature; common social and economic institutions; and either an existing independent government or plans for one. The psychological determinants include belief in a common history and ethnic origin, however consistent with the facts; regard for fellow "nationals"; devotion to what is called a nation; shared pride in its triumphs and grief for its defeats; common hostility toward other nations; and shared hope for the nation's security and prosperity in future.

Ethnonationalism

We assume that in man's prehistory the development of separate clusters of people gave rise to consciousness of differences between such groups. It seems that the major difference identified was the line of birth. Birth, lineage, and kinship feature prominently in consciousness of ethnicity and nationality. Ethnicity and nationality clearly have, or have historically had, some meanings in common as we observe their derivations from similar words and concepts, for example, a people, a breed, a race. We find the word *"ethnonationalism"* useful when referring to psychological processes common to "ethnicity" and "nationalism."

The recognition of a subjective psychological quality in ethnicity and nationalism is shared by other interested disciplines, such as political science, social psychology, and cultural anthropology, and is, in short, obvious. Other behavioral science disciplines deal with the matter at their own levels of observation and analysis. Psychiatric investigators at the interface of culture and psychiatry have studied the different expressions of psychiatric syndromes and their epidemiology in various cultures and ethnic groups and have been concerned with child-rearing and education. The field has shown little concern for the psychological development of cultural differences and has paid little attention to the larger ethnic context of human relations.

Ironically, ethnic and national data have a prominent place in identifying clinical cases. It is rare not to find a case description begin with such data as "A 40-year-old Irish Catholic carpenter. . . ." Implicit in this traditional approach to case identification is the idea that such data enable us to know something of the person. To do so we must, of course, call upon our own mental representations of the stereotypes of 40-year-old men, carpenters, and Irish Catholics. Stereotypes though chancy—nowadays we would have to stipulate the carpenter as male or female—are nevertheless embedded in our concept of the differences between groups. Ethnicity will not go away.

3

SOME THEORETICAL CONSIDERATIONS

In an earlier publication (GAP, 1978) our committee examined the way in which people experience their most intimate personal involvement in the nation's life in its most intense pitch, that is, in war.

We confirmed what has often been noted: National crises evoke from the individual strong feelings of participation in and identification with the national welfare. The psychological processes that underlie these phenomena are familiar to us from observations of small groups such as psychotherapy groups. However, certain phenomena (e.g., the merger of individual with the group) are intensified to an extreme degree by the life-and-death nature of war. Major national experiences and moods such as those of heroic grandeur and persecuted martyrdom echo and may bring into personal consciousness precisely analogous experiences and moods from each individual's early life. This heightening of personal consciousness is made possible in part by the favorable sanction of the group, which has the effect of suspending the critical faculties. The psychological material so activated and revived often appears to be drawn from the close-to-consciousness identification with great national figures who have served as role models during ethnonational education and enculturation. But much of the material is isomorphic with very early-life psychological positions of merger, grandiosity, and persecution, which psychoanalysis has been examining under the rubrics of object relations theory and self psychology.

The immediacy of involving the self with the group seemed to be most readily explained by psychoanalytic theories of narcissism and Kohut's self psychology. We commented (GAP, 1978):

> The sense of self as a mental content emerges gradually in the process of separation-individuation from a state in which the infant recognizes no distinction between it and mother. Its strength is so largely shared with or, rather, borrowed from the mother that impotent frustration prompts the emergence of a spectrum of regressive and aggrandizing maneuvers, including fantasies of delusional grandiosity and omnipotence and efforts at merger with idealized parents and other powerful images. Gradual taming and modulation via appropriate responses from the parents leads to an effective sense of worth and esteem, and even fuels ambitions and ideals in favorable development sequences. (p. 401)

In exploring the implications of narcissism for man's relationship to the nation in making war, we confined our efforts to a limited area of the field of object relations. The term *object relation-(ship)* is defined by Laplanche and Pontalis (1973) as

> a term enjoying a very wide currency in present day psychoanalysis as a designation for the subject's mode of relation to his world; this relation is the entire complex outcome of a particular organization of the personality, of an apprehension of objects that is to some extent phantasied. (p. 277)

Our clinical work readily persuades us of the difficulty in discerning what is objective and what is subjective in object relations. The truth is hard to find and is, and in the words of Laplanche and Pontalis, to some extent phantasied. In clinical psychoanalysis, as in the rest of life, the constant task is to winnow reality from fantasy. It is a life-long task, and some of the best of it is done later in life, a part of what Robert Butler (1975) has described as "life review."

While in the earlier work we studied those elements in the personality that are most immediately and consciously mobilized and brought to bear in pursuit of the group effort, the present work explores further the developmental foundations upon which this occurs. We see three foundations: biological; infantile psychological precursors of group belonging; and the establishment of ethnonational identity coincident with the crystalization of personal identity in adolescence.

We are increasingly impressed with the significance of biological forces in determining ethnonational behavior. Earlier we alluded to a spectrum of the degree of biological continuity between, and union of, the participants who comprise a community. The spectrum is represented at one end by certain marine species where the "unit" is not so much the individual particle as the colony and at the other end by species that appear to live with little social interaction, or, as in the case of man, consciously suppose more independence than the facts affirm. Evidence accumulates from various fields to suggest a closer and more complex relationship between biology, psychology, and social process. Perhaps human pride in human consciousness has slowed the integration of biology with psychology and social process. We cannot attempt a synthesis here, but any such effort would have to take man's evolutionary origin into account. Anthropologists offer valuable notions on the role of interpersonal and family attachments in the emergence of our species.

In lower animals mere physical mating and a limited repertoire of instinctually imprinted and learned nurturing behaviors suffice for the propagation of the species—but not for man. The evolution of the human forebrain required a complex system of human mating and parenting. The skeletal remains of early primates suggest to anthropologists that the archaic family had worked out a division of labor, with the male reliably sustaining his mate, who devoted herself to child-rearing, promoting the development of an increasingly intelligent brain throughout the long period of childhood dependency. The neuroanatomical and familio-social evolutions no doubt developed pari passu, each facilitating the other.

From the evolutionary standpoint forebrain growth and maternal care enjoyed a mutually reinforcing and positive feedback relationship. The intense interrelatedness of mother and child during the prolonged human childhood served to increase the child's ontogenetic ability to form intense human relations in later life. Increased psychological and social commitment between adult partners meant the emergence of the human capacity for being in love. From both evolutionary and ontogenetic standpoints the development during childhood of the ability to form and sustain strong human relationships spelled the emergence of a unique faculty. This was a faculty to form object relations that could be enduring and yet transferable, a portable faculty that held great potential for social organization.

Galanter (1981) has recently offered a sociobiological perspective on cohesiveness in large groups. He finds in Darwin's comments on the preening behavior of male birds the implication "that an underlying biological substrate of behavior might be transmitted through generations and might therefore fall under the influence of evolutionary adaptation" (p. 415). More recently animal ethologists have studied the role of "social releasers," which are biologically grounded signals for instinctual behavior. These are seen to work not only among individuals (e.g., in mating behavior), but also in large group behavior, such as in aggregations of bees. Such behavior has great adaptive value and is clearly of (unlearned) biological origin.

Kandel (1983) recently suggested that life experiences have the power to modify brain function by altering synaptic strength and regulating gene expression. He considers that the learning and unlearning of anxiety may involve long-term functional and even structural changes in the brain that result from alteration in gene expression. E. O. Wilson (1975), a leader in the field of sociobiology, has given consideration to the existence of operationally defined "conformer genes."

Galanter (1981) points out that "conformity to the group norms stands in many respects on the interface between religious ritual and subjective feelings of social cohesiveness" (p. 419). His studies of contemporary religious sects over the course of several years have convinced him that subjective emotional distress is inversely related to a person's feelings of affiliation with a large social group.

Further understanding of the ties between biology, psychology, and social behavior may be found in experimental psychology as exemplified in research on visual perception. The eye, despite some uncertainty about such matters as retinal biochemistry and the cortical interpretation of stimuli, has long seemed a pretty simple optical mechanism, rather like a camera. All scientists assumed that visual perception provides a veridical mirroring of external objects. But now, as Westlundh and Smith (1983) point out, "New Look" psychologists, using such techniques as the tachistoscopic fractioning method of presenting stimuli (usually pictures of people), at initially extremely quick and then successively prolonged exposure times, are struck by the motivational influences on perception, on what we "see." The data obtained, consisting of verbal reports and/or drawings by the subject of what he has seen, strongly suggest idiosyncratic attitudinal responses that are repetitive and unvarying for each individual. They are specific transformations of stimulus content that accord with the individual's usual psychological defense patterns of denial, isolation, projection, and so on.

Perceptgenesis, as the field is known, postulates that perception is not a simple mirroring of the object but that it entails "construction in the direction of the object."

> Percepts develop from potentiality to actuality, from stages of ambiguity with many condensed meanings to stages characterized by a single definite one. This description is not an addition of stimulus adequate details; rather it is a subtraction of individual-specific, subjective components. (Westlundh & Smith, 1983, p. 605)

The creation of the conscious percept is a dialectical process of construction between the world of objects and the individual's meaning system in that "the outer objects are referents of the percept; the psychologically effective stimulus is only constructed during the act of perception" (Westlundh & Smith, 1983, p. 606).

Work in this field is scientifically well founded, though quite experimental and hypothetical. Its pertinence to the clinical study of object formation has recently been explored (Kafka, 1983). Already there is evidence that certain universal psychological mechanisms such as projection and isolation arrive in a relatively fixed developmental sequence to exert their influence on perception. Further work may clarify the similarity between these formal characteristics of perceptgenesis and, a matter to which we shall shortly turn, Pinderhughes's formal universal influences (such as up as opposed to down; front against back; and light against dark) that program bias into all behavior.

The societal and narcissistic significance of "minor differences" between ethnic groups is a venerable concern in the study of ethnicity. Perceptgenesis now offers the prospect of widening the study. Studies of tachistoscopic responses to exposures of very short, medium, and long duration show patterns that are quite general. Very short exposure to a picture (e.g., a social scene) will produce very similar responses among a group of experimental subjects. Long exposure times will produce much more elaborate responses but still with a great similarity. But in the middle range of exposure times, a considerable variety of responses is obtained. These idiosyncratic responses represent the residue and influence of the individual's psychological development. In other words, the personal history, the instinctual life, and psychological defenses as well as current drive states determine the response, the percept.

The influence of drive states, affects, and the attention factor on perception is acknowledged. For example, a hungry subject sees more food on Rorschach cards than one who has just eaten. Family and social attitudes conveyed to the developing child may greatly influence his attention and hence his percept. Differential focus can subjectively shorten what is objectively longer exposure time and vice versa. Small objective differences may thus become large and therefore help explain the exaggerations and other distortions that characterize interethnic relations.

The experiments of Westlundh and Smith show how perception in process, with its own impulsive and defensive operations, leads to "moments" in which the perceptual product differs from individual to individual as well as to "moments" of great consensus. From these experiments we may learn how small objective differences enlarge subjectively, thereby advancing our understanding of the individual and group psychology of the narcissism of minor differences.

Certainly time is an important factor in interethnic relations; World War II GIs joked crudely that the longer they stayed in Samoa, the whiter the girls there became. The armchair humanist who has the luxury of time can come to share the rational consensus that "we are all more human than otherwise," but the traveler who actually rubs elbows with different ethnic groups experiences shorter or intermediate exposure times and often has idiosyncratic nonrational responses.

During the early years when instinctual and rational life are being brought into some variable degree of dynamic harmony, biological forces appear to shape much of what will in later life constitute an uneasy legacy of compromised thinking and world view. Psychoanalysts and anthropologists note the greater value that almost all societies place on light against dark, up against down, and right-handedness over left-handedness. Hamilton (1966) maintains that biologically determined aversion to feces contributes to prejudice against black people. Charles Pinderhughes (1982) offers a comprehensive set of hypotheses about ways in which universally occurring biochemical and physiological processes produce universally occurring mind sets regardless of the cultural context. This helps to explain why the essential core of ethnicity remains the same for the person and the ethnic group, whatever its personal and cultural vicissitudes may be.

Pinderhughes argues persuasively that paired but opposite physiological processes such as those underlying the parasympathetic/sympathetic dichotomy of the autonomic nervous system and the incorporative/excretory functions of the gut impose a corresponding dichotomy on mentation. Incorporative activities (primarily feeding, but also gazing, listening, touching, etc.) lead to object relations of the approach/affiliative/affectionate type. Excretory expulsion functions lead to object relations of the avoidance/differentiation/aggressive type. Pinderhughes calls these A-bonding and D-bonding respectively.

It appears that in very early stages of our object relations, we are

unable to achieve sophisticated ambivalent relationships and tend
simply to divide objects into those that are A-bonded and those
that are D-bonded. The former, in line with our theory of narcissism and understanding of paranoid processes, are aggrandized
and the latter renounced: "These processes are paranoid in the
sense that they produce false beliefs based on projections that ag-
grandize objects of identification and denigrate renounced objects"
(Pinderhughes, 1979, p. 35). Moreover, Pinderhughes sees groups
as having A-bonding not only between members, but also with
their common territory and belief systems, and D-bonding with
groups from which they are alienated. These reactions account for
what he calls "nonpathological group-related paranoias." We note
that though they may be group-adaptive and nonpathological for
the individual, they can be highly destructive in intergroup relations.

Pinderhughes's hypotheses are supported by his clinical experience with individuals and his studies of large social groups. Although
his work has not gone uncriticized, much of it has the ring of truth,
and many psychoanalysts can confirm elements of it from their
own clinical experience; still, more study is needed, particularly at
the group level. But the notion that the mental processes of adult
life continue to be influenced by their origins in neurological
development and the neurophysiology of early life finds support
from other sources, including the work of the baby watchers.

These observers—very much in the naturalist tradition but now
equipped with modern gadgets—have supplied data to confirm,
question, and sometimes refute the speculations of the theoreticians. The transformation of the newborn infant from a vegetative
and isolated entity to a rapidly interacting socializing participant in
the mother-child relationship is now being defined with greater
clarity, and evidence emerges to suggest that some stages of the
development occur even earlier than had been supposed. Some of
these social behaviors of the infant appear to emerge from, build
on, and supplant similar behavior that appears to be inborn and
automatic. An example of this comes from Emde and Harmon
(1972) who have observed automatic or "endogenous" smiling in
the newborn. This may originate in the brainstem, for it correlates

with other REM-related spontaneous behaviors and has been noted in the anencephalic. Maturation, of just a few to several weeks, brings a new kind of smiling that is a response to external stimuli of great variety. Further development, presumably the interaction with mother, brings an increasing selectivity to this exogenous smiling, which has a learned and interactive quality.

Though visual cues or stimuli have been extensively studied in this connection, there is increasing evidence that the other senses are active and important at very early ages. The various senses appear to have the faculty of interplaying with and substituting for one another in some respects. The study of different stimuli that elicit the same response forms the cornerstone of Heinrich Klüver's "Method of Equivalent and Non-equivalent Stimuli" (1936). The significance of these factors in the subsequent formation of the personality and the development of concepts of reality has been discussed by Kafka (1983) who makes the point that what experimental psychologists call object constancy (e.g., when a chair is seen to remain the same from whatever angle it is viewed) has implications for the psychoanalytic concept of object constancy (roughly, enduring love). Clusters of subjectively different stimuli that the individual sees and treats as "subjectively equivalent" are the building blocks of his psychological reality. Certain constellations of stimuli may lead to the formation of engrams, such as familiarity and strangeness, that are idiosyncratic for the person and his ethnic group. Thus, people may find comfort in their adult lives in the familiar blendings of sensory perception that identify their own ethnic group. It seems important to note the *blending* of sensory perception, since the process goes well beyond such simple visual perceptions as those of differences in skin color.

Brazelton, Koslowski, and Main (1974) studied the mother-infant interaction in the first 20 weeks of life and outlined not only such elements of reciprocity as looking intently, dull looking, looking away, touching, and speaking, but also their subtle modulation by both parties. It may be that the mother in "modeling" the infant induces patterns and rhythms of reciprocity that influence all later-life socialization. Brazelton reminds us of Watzlawick, Beavin, and Jackson's dictum "that it is impossible for two persons confronting each other not to interact and that one may speak of positive or negative interaction between two persons, but never of NO interaction" (p. 60).

Brazelton and colleagues (1974) noted the bimodal obligatory interaction of mother and child:

> No actor's behavior was ever independent of the expectancy of interaction. Each behavior, then, was either positive or negative in its 'intent' within this expectancy. It became important to attach an intentional significance to each behavior and cluster of behaviors, based largely on the context within which it occurred and the result it achieved in the sequential shaping of the interaction. (p. 60)

Much adult behavior remains under the sway of this prototypal pattern, even if the behavior is outside awareness or if every effort has been made to put the behavior aside. It may be useful to ponder whether confrontation between groups and between nations may similarly be captive to the compelling dialectic of bimodal obligatory interaction.

Presenting this heuristic proposition calls for a parenthetical paragraph on drawing parallels between large group behavior and early childhood behavior. It is a perilous passage, but not entirely without bridges. In addition to the persistence of some such behavior patterns from childhood into individual adult life, we note that these same patterns may be found in family life and in small group behavior. But it is quite probable that some of the mental mechanisms involved, projection and splitting for example, operate differently, and even for different reasons, in large group situations. Furthermore, in offering a developmental perspective, we recognize the influence of many other determinants of large group behavior—psychological, social, and economic, for example. There is abundant room for further exploration.

Let us now return to an aspect of early-life development that has great significance not only for the adult individual, but also for all individual and group socialization. The later developmental and evolutionary vicissitudes of inescapable interaction are too important to have been left to chance. Man's evolution required rituals. In discussing the ontogeny of rituals, Erikson (1966) saw the roots of the ritual in the mother-infant recognition phenomenon. This repetitive game fosters, we suppose, a sense of self in the infant and helps maintain it in the mother. It also prepares the infant for the spirit of unity with the mother that makes it possible to see any third party as other or intruder. The establishment of such boundaries of inclusiveness and exclusiveness is a prime function of ritual.

What we see here is the development of highly idiosyncratic and subtle ritual in the mother-infant dyad. In later development this ritual behavior will be utilized by the individual in interpersonal relations. This entails the growth of a mind set that is coopted by society for the conduct of each everyday encounter by means of subtle rituals that regulate greetings, speech, facial expressions, physical proximity, and so on. Beyond these largely automatic and unconscious rituals lie the formal rituals, such as those of religion and the rites of passage, which have long been of interest to anthropologists (see, for instance, Turner, 1977). In some respects ethnicity can be seen as a successor to religion as a social form for mobilizing sentiment; in other respects, one can regard religion as intensifying ethnicity. In either case, religion, like ethnicity, can be used to intensify group absolutes and increase group grandiosity.

Kafka (1983) in his discussion of ritual and ritualization has emphasized several of the boundary functions. Ritual is used to resolve what may be one of the greatest areas of conflict for the developing individual, that is, what is inside and what is outside? This is, in effect, to define the individual, to separate one biological unit from the mass that is the remainder of the species. Anthropologists in studying the rites of passage through which the individual becomes a "part" of his society are essentially dealing with social aspects of the same fundamental biological issue.

Since boundaries are a sine qua non in the formation of Erikson's species and "pseudospecies," the role of ritual is vital, at its worst causing simultaneous dehumanization, deanimation, and reification of the other and glorification and deification of the in-group. Successful benign ritual can celebrate the unique features of a group and the group identification of its members; such ritual defines the unit with some flexibility and tolerates others in a process that may be thought of as guarding against excesses arising from dehumanizing the other. Dehumanization is associated with driven, obsessive, inflexible ritualization, rigidity, and the adoption of absolute boundaries.

Rituals represent the condensed encounter of the material and psychological. Ethnic rituals are therefore of particular interest as signals of potential flashpoints of violence based on ethnocentrism. In addition to a quantitative monitoring of ethnic rituals, it may also be important to observe certain qualities, especially the precision of performance. Emphasis on the precision of performance of the ritual is an index of the spiritual charge with which the abstract elements invest the concrete symbols.

It is axiomatic that many nationalistic manifestations are quite irrational, even mad. During the Great War, for example, Englishmen and Germans, although fully aware of their kinship, believed that their fellow nationals were superior. Having the same religious faith, they prayed to the same God for support and the destruction of the enemy. And lest we in turn feel beyond folly, consider the race between the United States and Russia to obtain more than enough nuclear weapons to destroy each other 30 times over.

For intelligent, nonpsychotic people to hold such positions, a mental split is necessary—a special haven within the mind for mild madness, a place were one can reduce the rigors of rational thinking and indulge egotism, illusion, and fantasy. Here one can blend illusion and reality to taste, and say with Alice that the word means exactly what one wants it to. We have this mental twilight zone, and most of us are tacitly tolerant of it. As a generally accepted aspect of human frailty, it goes unchallenged.

This as an area of the mind is implied in little-noted parts of Winnicott (1953), who took as his place of departure the hypothesis widely held by psychoanalysts that the newborn experiences his main point of contact with the world, the breast, not as part of that outer world but as part of himself, since a reasonably good enough mother makes herself available and so sustains the infant's illusion. But only for a while. Inexorably, there is a transition to reality. The mother's inability to provide immediate gratification of all the infant's demands leads to a gradual relinquishment of the latter's solipsistic delusion. This highly narcissistic primary process mentation reluctantly yields to a recognition and acceptance of external reality. It needs time and some crutches to accomplish the transition, and even when it is accomplished, we know well from our psychiatric work with children and adults how strongly the primary process may reassert itself in times of stress.

The crutches an infant uses in the transition are usually thumbs or fingers to suck on, then pieces of sheets or blankets are introduced to the mouth. This infantile need is familiar to mothers and other caretakers who provide pacifiers or teddy bears. Since such objects are valuable as defenses against anxiety and depression, the wise parent tolerates them, accepting the baby's right to resort to such a compromise or transitional object, especially when tired or hungry. They usually are important to the child for a long time, often for several years, but as he becomes better able to manage reality, he abandons them.

The period of transitional objects is usually characterized by mumbling, babbling, imitating, and first attempts at speech and song, to which Winnicott applies the term *transitional phenomena.* These phenomena seem connected to early conscious experiences of the breast, oral feeding instincts, and other perceptions of the mother's body, hallucinations, and mnemic traces that represent "primary process" thinking. Only much later in human development do rational thinking and behavior largely supplant primary process mentation and behavior.

So, while agreeing with the traditional view of human nature as composed of an inner instinctual part and a rational part oriented to external reality, Winnicott claims room for a third experiencing part to which inner life and external reality both contribute. It is deeply intimate and idiosyncratic (only a certain blanket will do). He sees it "as a resting place for the individual engaged in the perpetual human task of keeping inner and outer reality separate yet interrelated" (1953, p. 90). It is an area of permitted illusion and in some form and degree persists into adulthood.

This formulation approaches and in some respects coincides with Freud's thoughts on the splitting of the ego in the defense mechanism of disavowal or denial. Using a case of fetishism for illustration, Freud (1940/1964) pointed out that an object (in reality) can be simultaneously recognized, affirmed, and yet be denied. Consciousness, caught and split between instinct and perception, manages to reconcile the inherent contradiction by the use of fetishes. 'Both of the parties to the dispute obtain their share; the instinct is allowed to retain its satisfaction and the proper respect is shown to reality" (p. 275). As Laplanche and Pontalis (1973) point out, the contradictory positions are not compromised but are maintained simultaneously and without the establishment of any dialectical relationship.

An analogous construct of contradictory elements may be at work in the ethnonational attitudes of the individual and the group. The inherent irrationality may be supported, in part, by the use of special group-shared fetishes. While fetishes are of course idiosyncratic and symbolic, they are also very real and comprise, in the case of ethnonationalism, such concrete objects as uniforms and flags. There may be a further and more metaphoric step in the process. Perhaps some words, ideas, and slogans, that have strong allusive and rallying qualities serve as fetishes to permit the suspension of reason for numbers of people, for the ethnic group.

The area of transitional mentation is seen by Winnicott (1953) as one from which art and religion may spring. It is a repository of highly personal quirks and eccentricities where wisdom has taught us not to intrude on one another. "We can share a respect for illusory experience, and if we wish may collect together and form a group on the basis of the similarity of our illusory experiences. This is a natural root of grouping among human beings" (p. 90). We suggest that these groupings do not occur only in the sense of organizing those scattered individuals who already hold certain illusory experiences and beliefs. Shared illusions are not the same simply by virtue of coincidence, but also by indoctrination. Families and society introduce their own beliefs and attitudes to this stage of the child's development. Although this stage is highly individualized and full of personal creativity, it is still quite malleable and susceptible to ethnic imprinting.

The Pinderhughes hypotheses offer a close fit with our knowledge of early object relations and with our extension of Winnicott's ideas on transitional phenomena and thinking. Inevitably, parents and their particular ethnic group introduce ideas into the growing child's education—many of them illusions of the "us-and-them" type—which are readily and uncritically incorporated by a mind in transition and receptive to ideas that conform to the innate tendency to dichotomize. The maturation of rational thinking modifies but does not completely eliminate the illusory thinking. It lies there only partly dormant and preconscious to be communicated endlessly to succeeding generations.

In biology, the term pseudophenomenon refers to a phenomenon that, although seemingly *sui generis,* is in fact a modification of a previously known entity. Erikson (1966) used the term pseudospecies in respect to the diversity of mankind. "Man has evolved (by whatever kind of evolution or whatever adaptive reasons) in pseudospecies, i.e., tribes, clans, classes, etc., which behave as if they were separate species created at the beginning of time by supernatural intent" (p. 61). Erikson speculates about the ways in which aggressive and sexual drives contributed to the clustering of human beings in certain well-defined groups.

Naked, upright, and unarmed, the human animal copied the better-armed lower animals by wearing their feathers or skins and feared humans from any other subspecies of mankind. Erikson notes that not only did each group develop "a distinct sense of identity, but also a conviction of harboring the human identity" (p. 606) and regarded others as "extraspecific and inimical to (genuine) human endeavor" (p. 606) Every newborn is a "generalist" creature able to fit into any pseudospecies, and it takes prolonged childhood for him to become "specialized."

If we are candid with ourselves, we acknowledge that we see

those of some other pseudospecies as inferior to ourselves, or bad; they provide a suitable screen for our projections of contempt, aggression, hatred, and so on. Pinderhughes (1982), discussing our differential aggressive bonding to such groups, calls them "common renounced targets," while Volkan (1986) calls them "suitable targets for externalization." Although love is considered an organizing force for the individual ego, so is hatred, and this may be true of society also. Ping-Nie Pao (1965), reviewing the ego-syntonic uses of hatred, wrote:

> Ernest Jones showed how hatred can serve to cover fear or guilt. Hill observed that it can serve to avoid 'feelings of dependency, of a need to be loved, of passivity and helplessness, or a desire to dominate and control (as a reaction-formation against passivity), and even feelings of affection.' Searles indicated that vengefulness or scorn can serve as a defense against repressed grief and separation anxiety. (p. 260)

Giving supporting clinical evidence, Pao asserted that "hatred may play an organizing and defensive role and may help to establish a sense of continuity and identity in the patient" (p. 263).

Jacobson (1964) studied how the concept of the self develops from those early infantile self-images that are our first body images and sensations and elaborated on the interaction between representations of the self and those of objects. Her attempt to understand psychotic patients led her to state that certain types of psychotic patients will not immediately break with reality but first attempt the opposite as Freud and Fenichel had proposed. She held that

> They try to turn to and to employ the external world as an aid in their efforts to replenish their libidinal resources, to strengthen their weakening ego and superego, and to resolve their narcissistic and instinctual conflicts with which their defective ego cannot cope .... They try to change it [the external world], to create one that will suit their special needs, and to reject and deny those aspects that are of no use to them. (pp. 18–20)

Although she did not elaborate on "normal" aspects of the attempt to change the external world and/or the perception and experience of it, she saw the psychotic patient trying to keep the cohesiveness of his self by influencing the external world; this view provides a starting point from which to explore the "normal" need to create an enemy in the external world (Volkan, 1985; 1986).

Speaking of the libidinal and aggressive cathexis of self- and object representations in the developing child, Jacobson described how libido and aggression are continually turned from the love object to the self (and vice versa), and/or from one object to the other, while certain images of the self and object fuse and separate again. She noted a tendency of the child not yet ambivalent-tolerant to cathect one group of self- and object representations with libido only and to invest another with aggression.

Kernberg's (1966, 1976b) widely known theory of internalized object relations emphasizes the bipolar building up of self- and object images (or representations made from more enduring collections of images) that reflect the original relationship of an infant and his mother. Kernberg then elaborated on the subsequent development of dyadic, triadic, and multiple internal and external interpersonal relations in general. In his early interaction with the mother (and of course other important care-givers, including father), the infant acquires his orientation to extrauterine life; pleasurable or disagreeable stimuli impinging on him make an ever-increasing number of memory traces on the inborn and autonomous-perceptive faculty of the primitive ego. From these, the individual forms in a bipolar way what Mahler (1968) calls "memory islands," which contain certain pleasurable (good) and painful (bad) stimuli not yet allocated either to the self or to the not-self. Through repeated experience with need-satisfying and need-denying outside sources, the infant develops self- and object images undifferentiated at first, but then separated along affective bipolar lines into "good" and "bad" units. Jacobson (1964) described "bad" units as tending to be invested with aggression and "good" ones with libido.

Kernberg (1976b) treats both self- and object representations as

affective-cognitive structures and believes that the early ego has two
basic tasks to complete in rapid succession: it must differentiate
self-representation from object representation and integrate libidinally
and aggressively determined self- and object representations. He
goes on to define the stages in which these tasks occur and to
describe with precision the clinical conditions and character pathology associated with fixation in each.

What interests us here is what happens when the child reaches
the age (usually 36 months) at which he can be expected to
complete the welding of his opposing good and bad units, along
with the opposing drive derivatives attached to each, in order to
achieve an integrated self-concept, integrated object representations, and more neutralized expression of the drives. Clinical
experience shows that such welding or mending is never complete,
and we do not refer to pathological fixations and such development as that of borderline personality organization (Kernberg,
1966), in which excessive splitting of opposing units is the dominant defense, but rather to the "normal" course of events. In this
phase the maturing ego, now more effective in repression, can
deposit in the child's id by repression unintegrated and unacceptable
parts of his primitive, internalized object relations, making part of
the id an "ego-id" (Kernberg, 1976b; van der Waals, 1952; Volkan,
1979). Moreover, the mending of opposing representational units
causes a feeling of "loss," in reaction to which the child establishes a
new set of idealized images. The coalescence of these into the
superego, which also contains unmended and excessively bad
images, integrates it and tames its ferocity.

Thus unmended good and bad self- and object images are
absorbed into the structures of mind, but the ego does something
else with them, and it is necessary to understand this as we search
for a solid link between individual depth psychology and group
behavior. The ego "normally" externalizes these units onto suitable
targets (Volkan 1985; 1986).

Externalization refers here to the developmentally normal and
adaptive mechanism by which the child puts into objects his
ego-dystonic parts, unmended self- and object images, idealized

self- and object images, and superego forerunners. Children do this playing with dolls and toys, often revealing a rich fantasy life as they invent heroes and villains in what is quite transparently an externalization of certain elements of their own lives and those of their families. The overuse of externalization in childhood indicates a defect in the ego's integrative functions. Projection, which is used to defend against a specific drive derivative directed at an object, develops later than externalization and can be used at a stage in which

> the capacity to manipulate objects in fantasy has developed to the point where a drive derivative originally directed at an object can be subjectively allocated to that object, while the self is experienced as the object of that drive derivative. In contrast to externalization of aspects of the self, which effectively do away with peaceful affect, projection may leave the subject a constant prey to anxiety. (Novick & Kelly, 1970, pp. 84–85)

It should be remembered that projection can, in later life, be condensed with externalizations (Volkan, 1979). A related phenomenon is Klein's (1955) projective identification, in which part of the self is split and projected onto another person with whom the individual then feels identified and who has become a reservoir of his own qualities.

Freud saw a grain of truth in paranoid projections, and Novick and Kelly (1970) speak of "some degree of fit" between what is projected and its target, noting that there may be only little fit between an externalized dystonic aspect of the self and the reality. For example, when a child falls, hurting himself, he externalizes his "fallen" (unacceptable) self onto a doll, which may not be a reasonable target but one the mother has suggested as a suitable receptacle for the child's still unmended units. Important others in the child's environment sponsor the selection of suitable targets for externalization.

A child's environment, furnished with people and things, is colored by mother-directed good and bad feelings (Searles, 1965).

As he distinguishes "others" from his mother, the latter plays a significant role in causing him to perceive some things as good and others as bad, her influence surpassing her child's experience and fantasies.

The familiar foods, odors, and sounds of the household or neighborhood in which he lives are suitable targets upon which a child can externalize aspects of himself. Shared by many in any given group, they constitute the building blocks that the children of that group will to some degree use throughout their lives in constructing and reaffirming their ethnic, cultural, or national identity. They may be "out there," but the child has invested something of himself in them, including raw feelings directed by early concepts of "me," "mother-me," and "mother." Those libidinally invested will support the cohesion of the self-representation that is retained; those invested with aggression will threaten it. Paradoxically, however, the latter when kept at a safe distance and contrasted with the good units will enhance the child's self-representation. Erikson's "generalist" is now a member of a pseudospecies, and although he may not acknowledge this in any sophisticated way, he will be able as he grows up to see himself as a member of a specific clan, ethnic culture, and nation.

The "suitable targets for externalization" symbolically given to children by like-minded important others make the children alike, although each child retains his own psychological individuality. At this point in their development it is these suitable targets that connect the individual with group psychology.

When Geertz (1973) and Shils (1957) speak as anthropologists and sociologists of "primordial ties," we believe they refer to the raw investment in the suitable targets of externalization. Such a tie is

> one that seems from the "givens"—or, more precisely, as culture is inevitably involved in such matters, the assumed "givens"—of social existence: immediate contiguity and kin connection mainly, but beyond the givenness that stems from being born into a particular religious community, speaking a particular language, or even a dialect of a language, and

> following particular social practices. These congruities of blood,
> speech, custom, and so on, are seen to have an ineffable, and
> at times overpowering, coerciveness in and of themselves.
> (Geertz, 1973, p. 259)

The network of primordial alliances (sharing the same suitable
targets for externalization) is usually the product of centuries of
gradual crystallization. Whether concrete (a national flag or national
cuisine, for example) or abstract (national identity or cultural
heritage), they can be studied from the viewpoint of history, econ-
omy, natural disasters, a leader's influence, and so on. The primary
contribution of psychoanalysis to this kind of study depends on the
fact that the targets contain elements of self-representations and
the attached raw drive derivatives. In normal times the adult accus-
tomed in childhood to such targets may be overwhelmed by their
intrapsychic importance, although he may have repressed any
memory of the mechanism that makes him feel furious when one
of his targets is attacked by another pseudospecies. The frequency
of such furious reactions is so great as to suggest the likelihood that
none of us is exempt from regression to primitive modes of psychological functioning. Splits into good-bad, overestimating the
value of "ours" versus "theirs," and structuring of social groups to
maintain these belief systems, may be inevitable, when circumstances are stressful, or when persons whom we endow as leaders
encourage—and themselves manifest—splitting and idealizing in
their manipulation of national systems and symbols (Bion 1961;
Devereux 1955; Dorn 1969; Kernberg 1976b; La Barre 1972; Rice
1969; Rioch 1970).

Anthropologists hold that sentiments derived from primordial
ties established in childhood are different from those less savage
ones based on ties developed in later life in more complicated
processes. Bonds of being white, Turkish, Jewish, and so on are
basic; those derived from membership in a club, a professional
organization, or a political party are secondary. People joined
together by such operational ties do not constitute a separate
nation on account of such bonding; only when they become

strongly enough infused with primordial emotions do they become sufficiently passionate to undermine the state itself. "Primordial discontent strives more deeply and is satisfied less easily" (Geertz, 1973, p. 26). The powerful emotional component of ethnicity is a subject we shall return to after examining the transformations that occur in adolescence, especially what happens to the targets of externalization.

Blos (1979) holds that a child has only character *traits* before character crystallization occurs in adolescence. The formation and crystallization is the end result of the ego's integrative work in the hope to avoid conflict and anxiety. Blos lists four preconditions without which adolescent character formation cannot take its proper course, calling the first "the second individuation." Anna Freud (1958) had observed that the adolescent loosens his ties to his infantile object representations (and corresponding self-representations). She discussed, as did Geleerd (1961) and Jacobson (1964) later, the regression of ego and superego that precedes the new integration required for the formation of character, which is phase specific in the promotion of development and encourages the adolescent to find objects of love and hate outside the family circle. According to Blos (1979):

> Adolescent regression in the service of development brings the more advanced ego of adolescence into contact with infantile drive positions, with old conflictual constellations and their solutions, with early object relatedness, and narcissistic formations. We might say that the personality functioning which was adequate for the protoadolescent child undergoes a selective overhaul. (p. 180)

This situation shifts the balance between ego and id. "New identifications ('the friends,' 'the group,' etc.) take over superego functions, episodically or lastingly" (Blos, 1979, p. 181).

Blos's second precondition is the conquest of "residual trauma" —residuals of conditions "unfavorable, noxious, or drastically injurious to the development of the young individual" (Greenacre,

1967, p. 277). These are assimilated in character formation and no longer cause repetitious signal anxiety.

The third precondition includes the corrective measures taken at adolescence to restore the integrity of the senses and reason, to correct "the family myth," and to accomplish continuity of the ego.

The fourth precondition that completes the set relates to the emergence of sexual identity. Blos agrees with many others in stating that gender identity is established at an early age whereas "sexual identity with definite, i.e., irreversible boundaries appears only belatedly as the collateral of sexual maturation at puberty" (1979, p. 186).

According to Blos, once all these preconditions are met,

> Character structure renders the psychic organism less vulnerable than it has ever been before, and the maintenance of this structure is secured against any interference from any quarter, internal or external. If must be, one dies for it before letting it die. (1979, p. 190).

However, Erikson (1956) notes that "identity formation . . . begins where the usefulness of identification ends" (p. 113).

Ego development after adolescence depends less and less on identification and permits the play of independent critical judgment and of individual autonomous trends of the ego and its anlage. Although the adult's sound development and self-realization depend on his being freed from the incestuous and dependent postures of his early life, his relationships and identifications with those important to him as a child are never altogether annulled. His ultimate identity will depend on the modification, stabilization, and integration of bygone relations and identifications and on his consequent ability to relate to and identify with groups in healthy and discriminating ways. The capacity to weave the realities of the past, however emotionally laden they may be, with those of the present makes for consistent and well-directed subsequent development in respect to emotional, sexual, and vocational aspects of life.

That is not to discount the significant influence on adult development exercised by relations and identifications with the group; but early loyalties stretch to include specific relations and identifications not only with his class and with the racial and national groups to which he belongs, but also with the vocational, social, political, scientific, or religious groups that he may decide to join. Since identification with and adherence to a group affects the individual's ego identity—his ideals, behavior, and social role—the individual with incompatible group identifications and relations usually experiences sharp identity conflicts, as demonstrated in clinical experience. Problems of protracted adolescence are evident in the narcissism, emotional lability, and need for validation that patients with conflicting group loyalties display. And even in high-level investment in the group, there remain raw investments from childhood that are echoed in such manifestations as ethnicity. When stressed, one's investment in ethnicity and adherence to the ethnic group outweigh any identification with a vocational, political, or social complex. Such formulations deal with what happens within the character or ego identity.

We now turn to what happens to the "suitable targets for externalization" outside, which are laden with elements from within, of which the individual is unaware. Volkan (1985) holds that although the prepubertal child is no longer "a generalist," his investment in his suitable targets is flexible until he goes through adolescence, when he would die for his good suitable targets before relinquishing them. During his second individuation (Blos, 1979), he reassesses them and strengthens his investment in some, abandoning it in others, being largely unconscious of doing so.

In normal adolescence the loosening of ties to internalized self- and object representations brings a mourning experience similar to that of an adult who has lost someone dear (Wolfenstein, 1966; Volkan, 1981). He then seeks new representations of self and object as replacements for what he has lost. These will be idealized at first, and some "bad" ones are psychologically pushed further away in order to safeguard those seen as ideal. Emerging from adolescence, the individual will tame his newly created self- and object representations by a process of integration. However, the mourning process that accompanies adolescent overhauling, with its rejection of unsatisfactory infantile representations and the taming and integrating of newly created self- and object representations, is never entirely complete, just as the "normal" welding of opposing good and bad self- and object representations falls short of completion.

"Suitable targets" are now chosen in accordance with the views of the peer group rather than under the mother's direction, although early parental influence does persist in some degree. The postadolescent is apt to rediscover under group pressure most of the originally mother-directed targets that were based on primal sentiments, although they may now be disguised or called by different names. As his horizons expand beyond his family and neighborhood, he observes the world at large from a new point of view. Familiar objects such as flag, food, language, and skin color continue to provide material for externalization, but now abstract conceptualizations infused with affect such as ethnicity appear, and he accepts them as even more suitable targets for externalization. Ego identity (Erikson, 1956) has an intimate affective relationship with such suitable abstract targets; the concept of self and that of the suitable targets are intertwined. Any appreciation of the value of a good target increases the individual's self-esteem, and an attack on his ethnic group reduces it. Although ego identities differ from one to another within the group, its members share the same good and bad targets, and these glue them together. Later we will discuss other binding factors such as devotion to the same leader.

The absorption of residual trauma into character, Blos's second precondition for adolescent character formation, is not wholly accomplished. When there is pathology,

> Those adolescents who sidestep the transformation of residual trauma into character formation project the danger situation into the *outside world* [emphasis added] and thus avoid the internal confrontation with it. By having failed to internalize the danger situation, the chance for coming to terms with it is forfeited; projecting it at adolescence onto the outside world

results in a state of apprehension over victimization; indecision and bewilderment ensue. (Blos, 1979, p. 184)

What Blos refers to are not externalizations of unmended self- and object representations but projections of dangerous situations stemming from mental conflicts. When the externalization of self- and object representations and projection of dangerous situations onto the same targets are condensed, this makes the targets psychologically indispensable. Through these processes, things "out there" are linked to ourselves (Jaffe, 1968). Although the state Blos speaks of above is exaggeratedly pathological, we think that such projections occur "normally" when sanctioned by other members of the group who use the same targets for their projections.

What is true of Blos's second precondition can be seen in his third also. Although the adolescent ego tries to establish "historical continuity," continuity is established to a "normal" degree by projections and externalizations of suitable targets, some dystonic aspects, or drive expressions, which other members of the group share. As the adolescent establishes a sexual identity, the "sexuality" of his targets is seldom a determinant of their selection, since either men or women of one ethnic or racial group can become targets for the reception of "good" or "bad" unmended self- and object representations from members of another.

The emotions of ethnonationalism, unmistakable and intense, are gut feelings of love and hate that give ethnicity its color and force. The sense of belonging to a group is an intimate part of the sense of self. Associated with this are deeply experienced subjective feelings and attitudes concerned with self-esteem, trust of others, and basic worries over safety and survival. To understand these aspects of ethnicity, one must grasp how affects develop and interact with early and subsequent self-object relations.

The emotional roots of ethnicity lie in affects attached to it in all phases of life, but particularly those connected with experiences and object relations of very early life. Sandler and Sandler (1978), Krystal (1974, 1975), and Krystal and Raskin (1970) provide useful insights for understanding the way affects attach to ethnicity and govern its quality and manifestations. The former expand and clarify Winnicott's ideas that help explain how early object relations and their extension into adult life influence basic affect states and affiliative tendencies. They suggest, in contrast to Winnicott's focus on the satisfaction of instinctual drives, that wishes or needs about significant objects are not so much derived from instincts as from a need to restore a sense of well-being and safety. They emphasize that such needs involve "wished-for interaction" with objects that provide "nourishment—affirmation and reassurance" —and note that a sense of safety and reassurance comes from unconscious dialogue with our objects in fantasy, and that people try to realize current dominant unconscious desires for well-being and safety. The attempt to actualize wishes or needs takes many forms, but "illusional" and "symbolic" actualization seems to come close to how one's sense of belonging and identity through one's ethnicity serves the purpose and "makes actual" a sense of well-being and safety.

The Sandlers' observations of how certain needs are revealed in group process comes close to capturing how ethnics make use of and draw comfort from group identification.

> Members of a group will "negotiate" with one another in terms of the responses which each one needs and in terms of the responses which are demanded of him. The members of the group may even make unconscious "deals" or "transactions" in terms of the responses involved so that each gains as much object-related wish-fulfillment as possible in return for concessions to other members of the group. (1978, p. 291)

Krystal and Raskin (1970) and Krystal (1974) have postulated a developmental line for affects from less mature to more mature forms. Krystal's conceptualization provides a helpful basis to explain developmentally some of the qualities of intensity and variability with which affects become attached to ethnicity. He has postulated that affects at the outset are undifferentiated, somatized, and not verbalized. The normal thrust of development is in the direction of differentiation, desomatization, and verbalization, and, as with other aspects of mental life, affects are subject to developmental arrest and traumatic regression.

Krystal (1974) cites the work of Schmale (1964), who described how the earliest experiences of pleasure and unpleasure with primary objects result respectively in feelings of bliss and helplessness. Subsequently, with differentiation of object and self, the development of motor skills, and the acquisition of speech "self-initiated" activities evoke either approval and gratification or disapproval and guilt. Accordingly, the child learns early that initiative may bring either pride or shame. Schmale notes that as the child becomes aware of the possibilities and vicissitudes of exercising self-control, he practices the living out and handling of pride and shame. The qualities of such affects and the objects to which they become attached may transfer in later life and become attached to attitudes about ethnicity.

Krystal repeatedly underscores the importance of desomatization and verbalization as ways of mastering affect. He suggests that the use of any kind of symbol or image may promote desomatization, thus affects and object relations may develop and attach themselves to attitudes about ethnicity along a number of continuums of immature to mature expression. Such continuums might, for example, include the nonverbal-verbal, concrete-abstract, irrational-rational, and crude-refined.

Such formulations about the role of affects in relation to ethnicity represent only a preliminary attempt to explore some of its developmental and intrapsychic underpinnings. What seems to be so different among various ethnic groups turns out, upon examination, to be only differences in shade, coloring, and form of universal human phenomena. The uniqueness of ethnic experience depends on packaging rather than on substance or content. All ethnics share a need for security and comfort, face problems of human suffering and repair, are challenged by separation and maturation, and experience pride and shame. Ethnicity often becomes a convenient way of expressing or mastering characteristically human struggles and conflicts. For example, one is reminded of the nostalgia and romanticism about "the old country" expressed by many ethnics; although so many emigrated because of cruel and oppressive realities, they cling to happy memories and feelings for their homeland. One might suspect that much of the strength and sustenance ethnics obtain from their national origins comes from the quality of early unambivalent ties to significant objects that transfer to ethnic themes and provide a comforting, secure source to draw upon, no matter how harsh or traumatizing one's realities become in later life.

It is also evident that affects attached to ethnicity may produce problems in adaptation. The "problem" of affects in relation to ethnicity is not that ethnicity is laden with affect (which is true enough), but that the affects attached to it are often primitive, undifferentiated, and vague, unmodified by the taming and moderating influences of reflection and reason. This explains why interethnic relations are so notoriously subject to primitive processes and psychological mechanisms such as externalization, projection, projective identification, splitting, and distortion.

We must acknowledge in closing this chapter that our understanding of the metapsychology of ethnicity is tentative, theoretical, and incomplete, leaving much room for additional and differing observations and judgments. Is it normal or abnormal? Good or bad? As our committee studied the role of cultural and ethnic elements in the psychological development of the individual, two different views emerged—and were not reconciled.

One view holds ethnicity to be a normal aspect of development. The growing child's ego deals with the everyday sights, sounds, smells, and tastes of his culturally colored environment as natural, normal components of a system of internalized (mental) representations of the external world. His culture and ethnicity become both metaphorically and literally part of him; they are thoroughly ego-syntonic. Differences, whether large or small, can then be seen as simply a different set of sensory stimuli having their own cultural significance. Differences need not be thought of as abnormal, and repudiation of an alien culture is not necessary; differences can be transcended by empathic understanding. By analogy this view corresponds to Kohut's (1971) contention that there is a "normal" narcissism.

In the other view, ethnicity is regarded as being at least quasi-pathological, much as Kernberg considers narcissism. Again the developing ego is seen as having to establish an inner-object world from the essentials that the senses perceive. In the process and as contact occurs with other cultures, there is a tendency to seize upon and utilize the differences in order to compensate for and alleviate some of the developmental problems the ego may be having in other areas, for example, differentiating self from mother. In this view a displaced or retrospective use is made of ethnic differences and the quasi-pathological processes involved cause minor differences to be elevated to the status of significant differences—with many personal and social consequences.

We can learn from our apparent impasse. All theories, including those about human nature, are colored by the terrain being explored and the ideological needs of the explorer. We are no exception. How we deal with our own ethnicity helps determine what theories we find most congenial and how we develop and invest in them. Avoiding either extreme of optimism or pessimism about ethnicity, we keep open minds about whether it can be a positive, integrating influence on culture without becoming a malignant force that tears mankind apart.

4

THE INDIVIDUAL AND HIS ETHNICITY

Here we discuss how theory as outlined in the preceding chapter affects an individual's sense of ethnicity and national identification. There is no lack of material interpreting the accompanying phenomena in terms of such familiar concepts as oedipal issues, paranoia, and sibling rivalry. Although we acknowledge basic and valuable insights in this literature, we feel that progress in psychoanalysis and sociology, as well as our own observations, have enlarged our understanding. We have become aware of many mutually reenforcing dynamic processes that account for the great variety of ethnonational experiences.

Although we hypothesize here that a certain set of psychodynamics concerned with boundaries, both personal and interpersonal, promotes a sense of ethnicity and nationalism, we acknowledge that it can produce other social attitudes and divisions as well.

Irene Fast (1979), in discussing the psychology of gender identity and differentiation, goes beyond Freud's statement that "anatomy is destiny," pointing out that early realization of differences in sexual anatomy is followed by the awareness that one is either male or female and must abandon any sense of omnipotent totality—a discovery that often causes hurt and rage. Discomfort over this limitation may appear in something as innocent as same-sex conversational clustering at a party or as virulent as the exploitation of women by men that is customary in so many societies.

We recognize too the impact of social and economic forces on individual and family development. Considerations such as scarce resources—often associated with large families—can have a powerful society-wide influence on individual development, even to the

extent of producing patterns and stereotypes. We would not disa-
gree with Yeats (1959) who put it pithily:

> Out of Ireland have we come.
> Great hatred, little room,
> Maimed us at the start.
> I carry from my mother's womb
> A fanatic heart. (p. 249)

Yeats was of course writing at a time when Ireland's social problems
were still being compounded by overpopulation, the bitter aftermath of the Great Famine, and emigration. But the Irish, no less
than others of the world's poor, are noted for a contrasting willing-
ness to share their crust of bread. This coexistence of hatred and
generosity is another testimony to the resilient ambivalence of the
human spirit.

The operational field of the individual's ethnonational psychodynamics is so extensive that we must confine ourselves here to
sampling three areas. First, we review the way growing children
come to identify themselves and others in ethnonational terms.
Next, we present some case vignettes to illustrate the links between
theory and clinical practice. The final section of this chapter deals
with the dynamics of the leader and the group. Our consideration
of this significant relationship then introduces a chapter on intergroup dynamics.

Ethnicity in Children

It may be interesting to review briefly what behavioral sciences
other than psychoanalysis have to say about ethnicity in the development of children.

Mary Ellen Goodman (1964), a cultural anthropologist, deals
with race awareness in young children. She tells of several children
of three or four asking such questions as "What am I?" in clear
reference to their skin color. She feels that by the age of three the
child is conscious of self and has a growing sense of others and his

separation from them. New internal psychological percepts arise as a result of change and growth, although they have continuity with past experiences and psychological development. Furthermore, the past becomes transformed to provide important counterforces for the current new balance of psychological percepts. Children's language acknowledges the boundaries separating mother, father, siblings, and playmates from the personal self. Coming to see oneself as autonomous and separate from others is both exciting and painful, and this may account for the repetitive evidences of a search to identify the group to which one belongs. This is a recurrent and often lifelong theme. The individual tests boundaries of his own and of the groups around him, seeking feelings of safety and security to offset his awesome autonomy.

Goodman offers many examples of four-year-olds exhibiting curiosity and an ability to clearly identify, describe, classify, evaluate, and compare themselves to others. Their drawings reflect awareness of such things as gender, age, personal characteristics, family roles, and clothing. She did her field work on the East coast with 103 four-year-olds in a nursery school. Fifty-seven of these were defined socially as "Negroes" although they were not alike in color, hair, or features. The other 46 children were labeled "white"; they ranged from blond to brunette, from being light-skinned to dark-skinned, and indeed some were more heavily pigmented than their "Negro" counterparts. The neighborhood was a melting pot, people of various national origins and races having lived together for many years. Both sets of four-year-olds were aware of color and its meaning in varying degrees. Goodman divided both "Negro" and "white" children into those of low, medium, and high awareness. Of the 57 Negroes, nine were not often aware of their differences, but 26 were. Twenty-two were sensitive and aware most of the time. Among the 46 whites, seven were but faintly aware, 28 aware some of the time, and 11 seldom overlooked the difference.

An important finding, but one that needs further research, deals with superiority-inferiority dealing among four-year-olds. Interestingly, the white children never indicated feeling that blacks were inferior. A kind of lukewarm midpoint on the superiority-inferiority continuum does appear frequently. About half the white children seemed to feel nothing more marked than a passive neutrality, but the rest felt close to the superior end of the scale.

In contrast, the black children felt superior only to one another and never did they assume a posture of superiority toward whites. They did not manifest the subtleties of expression that spell superiority orientation among whites. Forty percent expressed neutrality, but over half the black children conveyed a sense of being inferior to whites.

Goodman (1967) later pointed out how uniquely individual most children's reactions to the wide range of cultural possibilities are, enculturation being a complex process. Somehow children make their own choices from the wide range of options open to them or recommended to them. Her work and that of Thomas, Birch, Chess, Hertzig and Korn (1963) indicate that children are highly adaptable and can cope with a wide range of opportunities. Despite inborn uniqueness, children in the same learning situation become more and more alike since learned behaviors soon overlie differences. It seems reasonable to suppose that perceptions of differences accountable for ethnicity have very early roots and are clearly quite distinct by the age of four in respect to cognition, affect, and sensorimotor activity.

McDonald's (1970) research on ethnicity was based on work in a therapeutic nursery school and kindergarten attended by white and nonwhite (black, Oriental, and Indian) children. She speaks specifically about "skin color anxiety." Like Spitz (1965), she noted that the smiling response disappears after the age of six months, the infant reserving his smiles for mother and other familiar persons after that. She called eighth-month stranger anxiety "the first manifestation of *anxiety proper*," considering it, like Spitz, a recognition of the mother as a separate person of specific importance.

She tells of one 10-month-old black baby who cried "desperately" with a white visitor but settled happily with any of the blacks in a strange household, permitting them to hold and care for her. In a footnote she gives two other examples, both regarding white babies— one frightened by a dark-skinned Mexican and the second, 12 months old and "past the peak of his stranger anxiety," who "screamed and shrank away in terror at his first contact with a dark-skinned African student from a nearby university" (p. 33).

McDonald follows the psychoanalytic terminology and concepts widely known because of Edith Jacobson's work on object relations, Phyllis Greenacre's study of identity, and Anna Freud's investigation of development, especially that of developing object relations. McDonald believes the child begins developing his first sense of identity, body boundaries and appearance, and separateness from mother at 12 months of age and regards skin color as an important and confusing factor at that time, correlating it with ego development and the establishment of body boundaries and image.

She gives interesting examples of the confusion of anxiety about skin color with developmental experiences and of conflicts of the oral phase with dislike for food of a given color. She tells of a boy angry over being brown, who seemed frightened that his teeth could turn brown too; she sees this as associated with his anger, possibly punishment for his angry outbursts over his hated color. An Oriental boy was very angry at the news that his mother was going to have a baby. There were both toileting and eating problems as he displaced his angry feelings from the expected infant onto a black friend, saying that the boy's tongue was brown. McDonald notes how the minority child of two or three handles feelings of inferiority by turning passive into active, rejecting the white child before he himself can be rejected.

McDonald thinks therapeutically, pointing out that dark minority children can achieve a positive sense of self-esteem though not without much more effort than the white child. They remain sensitive and vulnerable to stress and conflict. Their self-esteem can return, but a new child in school is a challenge, especially if white; feelings of self-devaluation and fears of being unwanted come back.

If children notice skin-color differences in the first year of life, we-they polarizations may occur at the same time that object constancy develops. These processes may reinforce each other as clinging-love focused on to the "us" maternal figure and group and as fear and rejecting-anxiety directed out onto the "them" individual-other and group.

Well before the oedipal period, dyadic relationships shift to include others as the soundly developing child demonstrates the ability to merge with and feel secure in the social "we" group. It symbolizes and further supports a positive sense of the self as a separate and valued individual. The child who feels small, helpless, and weak compensates by believing more and more in what he can accomplish with the help of the family. By the oedipal phase he should be assertive and confident, instead of envious and scornful, now being able to enjoy his body and its functions and to have a core body image and intact identity. Autonomy and mature interrelatedness are not contradictory in the context of early awareness of differences. Though a person's state is the product of the first 18-24 months of life, other persons have helped form the sense of self. A balance between autonomy and dependence is struck.

Should the preoedipal years be heavily colored by an overabundance of attachment, separation anxieties and ambivalence, skin-color problems with their inherent predispositions, further augment and reinforce the castration anxieties and concerns of the oedipal period. In these instances, the Oedipus complex of the boy and the girl child may not be resolved as nuclear family issues. It may remain, predisposing to primitive defenses, suspiciousness of others, and failures to resolve oedipal issues in a timely and appropriate fashion. Marmor (1966) has commented about people who fail to resolve the Oedipus complex: "They remain uneasy with strangers, and are able to love only people who are like themselves. . ." (p. 218). He goes on to explore the social and international consequences of this personal immaturity.

A comprehensive work on the literature on child ethnicity has been provided by Proshansky (1966). Starting with the work of Clark and Clark (1947), Goodman (1964), and several others, he also concludes that both white and black children show evidence of racial awareness by age three, and that this is firmly established as part of their perceptual psychic structure by the time they enter school. He believes that awareness of religious and national differences, which are, after all, less visible, do not appear until children begin to attend different churches and talk about differences in nationality and, perhaps, in dress.

Hartley, Rosenbaum, and Schwartz (1948), in working with children between the ages of three and 10, found membership in an ethnic minority to predispose to early development of ethnic awareness. Radke, Trager, and Davis (1949), in working with Jewish children between the ages of five and nine, described their being more strongly identified with their own ethnic group than Catholic or Protestant children, just as Goodman (1964) had found Negro children more racially "aware" at an earlier age than white children.

Proshansky differentiates an ethnic orientation from an ethnic attitude, the former having been described by Goodman (1964) as an "incipient attitude." Roughly between the ages of four and eight, children acquire a vocabulary and concepts reflecting ethnic attitudes, and these appear in their speech. Like sexual language, children's outspokenness about differences is modified by the attitudes of adults toward it. Children seldom grasp the full meaning of dubious ethnic terms; the ability to generalize, to comprehend fully, and to select terms appropriate for one's feelings comes with age and social experience.

Radke and associates (1949) are the only researchers to provide data on very young children's acceptance or rejection of those of another race, religion, or nationality; this is, however, usually a lively issue by age seven or eight, when hierarchies of values and class are evident in peer and school activities. Authority then shifts from the family to teachers and others in respect to much of the child's life, and the latency child has many social reenforcers. Investigators agree that prejudicial attitudes can begin by the age of six, although it takes many years for them to become full-blown through the processes of differentiation and integration in grammar and high school.

Young children are often threatened by tales of "bad children" being taken away from home by gypsies or other unknown persons. As in fairy tales, they make room for the dichotomizing of ambivalence; the child soon learns that gypsy life has its attractions, and when angry, he may threaten to run away and join it. The adolescent often transfers his allegiance to "different" groups and even to exotic cults. In the life of school and neighborhood, the dangerous representations are discovered in the "stranger" and the "foreign family."

Cross-cultural studies on ethnicity in childhood are now beginning to appear. Powell (1983) provides five contemporary articles particularly rich in additional cultural and ethnic data about the first five years of life. Research on black children in America is reported by Norton (1983), on Mexican-American by Mejuia (1983), on Filipino-American by Santos (1983), and Korean-American by Yu and Kim (1983). Although all the latter works are consistent with the general thrust of our work, we find that Powell's broader cross-cultural data base makes her book unique. An article by Romero (1983) warrants attention since, in a very constructive way, he points out shortcomings of both infant and preschool research accomplished to date and makes many suggestions for future investigation of physical, social, and symbolic environments during the first 12 years of life.

It seems evident from all this literature that the infant can begin between eight and twelve months of age to discriminate between the familiar other with whom he associates as "we" and others whom he anxiously experiences as "they." Such discrimination accounts for awareness of racial differences in the three-year-old toddler. Between the ages of four and seven, children verbalize their increasing awareness of racial and ethnic differences and similarities. Thus we suggest that according to the findings of Goodman and Proshansky, *ethnic orientation* is a useful term to designate growing ("incipient") attitudes that appear between the ages of four and eight years. Differences in skin color, being clearly visible, are noticed by children between the ages of three and four, and differences in nationality by those between five and eight. The term *ethnic attitudes* could then be reserved for the gradual structuring and integrating of adolescence that reach completion in adult life. Cross-cultural studies appear to substantiate the psychological, anthropological, and psychoanalytical findings we have discussed.

Ethnicity in the Adult: Case Vignettes

In this section we explore some of the ways in which the metapsychology of the preceding chapter manifests itself in the adult.

The committee evaluated psychological material from literature, biography and autobiography, and interviews with the studies of untroubled individuals whose personalities their ethnicity has helped shape. But above all, as professionals whose interest in ethnicity was quickened by our committee's assignment, we shared our clinical experience. The psychoanalytic background of the majority of the committee permitted the examination of much material on each of the many cases we studied. The presentation here of material from clinically distressed people in whom issues of ethnicity were prominent should not be understood to equate ethnicity with psychopathology.

We carefully reviewed the psychoanalytic data that tie the theory we have presented to those aspects of individual behavior that may be called ethnonational. However, we will not here attempt the kind of detailed psychodynamic account more appropriate for a psychoanalytic journal, giving only vignettes that illustrate the daily influence of ethnonational identity and its clinical vicissitudes on personal life. To honor confidentiality we have condensed and disguised the cases reported and use fictitious names.

Many people accept ethnicity unselfconsciously as a natural part of their lives, an aspect of the prevailing culture they feel no need to examine or question. This is perhaps particularly true for members of homogeneous populations, and for the members of a majority or dominant group in a heterogeneous one. But even in such groups there are many for whom ethnicity is a significant element in personality formation, and social upheaval—and certainly war—stirs the sleeping dogs of ethnicity in almost everyone.

It must be emphasized that ethnicity is a cogent factor in minority groups, especially when they have long suffered social inequality and injustice because of it. The white/black dichotomy of American society has produced not only enormous social pathology, but much personal conflict. In our clinical work we have been greatly struck by the depth and importance of the personal factors underlying what presents clinically as "merely" ethnic or cultural. Behind such stereotypes as "black male" and "Jewish mother" we find poignant personal experiences of formative and transformative intensity.

Vignette 1

Our first story illustrates how the light/dark and black/white distinction in an American black influenced her perception of and feelings toward a fellow black of light pigmentation, and how in turn such ethnic distinctions were bound up with her sense of self-worth. A black female resident in family practice was called late at night by her hospital's emergency room to see a black man in his twenties who had cut his wrists lightly in a suicide gesture. After she admitted him, she found herself feeling increasingly annoyed at him, and resentful. She made hostile and scornful remarks to him without knowing why. She asked her supervisor, "Couldn't he at least have made a *real* suicide attempt? This one was so feeble! Anybody getting me out of bed had better do-himself-in good!"

Although her hostility was partly due to having been called out at night when very tired, a more important cause came to light in her supervisory sessions; the suicide attempt had reactivated anger toward her dead husband, who had shot himself some years earlier. Moreover, her skin was almost blue-black, but her husband had been, like the patient who so annoyed her, light-skinned. She called them both "pretty boys," explaining that this was a term used by blacks for those of their kind whose comparative pallor was thought to convey advantage in the world of white people. As she talked, she realized that she "saw" her husband in many attributes of her patient: keen intelligence, manipulativeness, depressiveness— and now the parallel of self-destructiveness. It was as though in this countertransference, which she recognized only slowly, she had to face her husband's death anew. Rather than be haunted by his memory and the separation panic she had repressed, she reacted by resenting the patient. Over the course of several consultations, she gradually became able to differentiate between the representation of her husband and that of the patient and was simultaneously able to see something she liked about the latter.

A decade or so earlier, she participated in the "Black Consciousness" movement of the late 1960s and early 1970s, and her African origin and blackness became a vitally important part of her identity. Yet during the years of her premedical and medical education she had sought the company and intellectual stimulation of whites, many of whom were Jews. As the supervisory consultations progressed, her countertransference toward the patient gradually lifted, and a transference toward the consultant appeared and consolidated. She now found in her supervisor, a Jewish man, many of the failings she had found in the patient. She vacillated between admiration and envy, seeing him as an asset to her clinical training and as utterly superfluous; as an ally in the department and an adversary obstructing her education; and as all-wise and as someone with nothing to contribute to blacks. She accused him at times of doing nothing right, but at other times, even in the same conversation, she would praise him for doing everything right. In short, idealization rapidly alternated with denigration.

She gradually came to realize that she especially resented the favored status the light-skinned enjoyed among blacks as well as among whites; she associated such status with whiteness and Jewishness and maleness in general, and with the consultant in particular. She externalized her sense of degradation and worthlessness onto her consultant, doing to him what she felt the patient had wrongfully done to her. In this way she was temporarily able to regain her sense of self-worth and to associate it exclusively with blackness, but that quickly troubled her, for she also did not want to lose what she had just repudiated in the consultant. She wanted access within herself to aspects she associated with blackness and whiteness. Ethnicity became for her, at least in part, an outer stage on which she enacted—and now tried to understand—an inner drama of ambivalence.

Her transference to her supervisor clarified her countertransference to the patient. She verbalized her envy of her dead husband, the intelligence and opportunities she wished had been hers. She did in fact have them within her, but denied them to keep her from feeling guilty for aspiring and succeeding among whites as a dark-skinned black. By holding that these images "belonged" to her husband, she could not only preserve her contempt for her husband and herself, but also her tie with the former, whose death she had been unable to mourn because of anger. She made personal and professional progress as she worked through these feelings of anger, which, although highly personal, were heavily cloaked with ethnic issues.

Vignette 2

This case illustrates an antithetical evolution, one in which the family ethnicity is rejected. Here ethnicity is not transcended in favor of a higher ideal, but, on the contrary, is sufficiently intense to account for what amounted to a lifelong imposture.

A 60-year-old physician sought psychiatric treatment for increasing anxiety and depression that made him drink to excess. His symptoms were recent and quite disconcerting as he had hitherto been successful and well disciplined. After completing his medical education in his native city, he had begun practice in a city several hundred miles away and quickly established himself. A good public image was important to him; he made the most of his blond good looks, Anglo-Saxon name, athletic ability, and membership in the Episcopal Church.

Though his manner was poised and persuasive, he had some undesirable personality traits, being rather deliberate and a bit too controlling with his patients, who considered this as evidence of his interest in them. Few saw that behind his facade he was actually quite dependent on them. To his wife and son he appeared to be domineering and demanding, but the former finally recognized the dependency he could not himself acknowledge. She herself was very dependent and reared their children with some difficulty; when they left home, she stopped trying and lapsed into using alcohol and tranquilizers, which her husband supplied. In an effort to save herself, she finally left him and got along better without him. His clinical problems began when he was left alone.

His public personality was designed to disguise what he thought of as his problem—he was Jewish. His father was a successful but striving professional, and his mother also was never content, always demanding more from her family—"typically Jewish—pushy and possessive"—he said. "She was a teacher and very controlling. I couldn't wait to get away from home." As a boy he had been "fat and ugly, so ashamed I'd never get into a swimsuit."

Feeling overfed, feminized by his mother, and too fat, he reacted in high school by becoming athletic, remaining so all his life. After medical school he distanced himself from his family psychologically and socially as well as literally, but was clearly unable to escape his dependency on his mother, his denial of it, and his controlling nature. He made no attempt to analyze the reason for these troublesome traits, but stereotyped them as being Jewish and ascribed them to his mother. He used Jewish ethnicity to deny and externalize parts of himself he hated, and adopted WASP ethnicity to achieve and support his ego ideal.

His personality conflicts were his ultimate undoing. The main artery of one leg became so constricted that he had to abandon his vigorous games of handball, so he had surgery to correct it. He foolishly began playing handball again too soon after the operation, and the artery ruptured and his leg had to be amputated. "I should have known better," he mourned. His image was shattered; he saw himself as flawed, ugly, weak, childish, and feminine. Becoming dependent on drugs and alcohol, he died in circumstances that suggested suicide.

Vignette 3

In contrast to this tragic imposture is the case of a gentile who tried to cope with feelings of confused identity by embracing the Judaism in which he was reared. His attempt at a sublimated solution was not entirely successful, and symptoms of depression brought him to psychotherapy when he was 25. His parents had divorced when he was three. His mother remarried a Jew when he was five and allowed her son to be reared as a Jew although she herself was not Jewish. The boy was sent to Jewish parochial schools, where he excelled. The other boys noticed at gym classes and at summer camp that he was not circumcised and made fun of him. Circumcision became an important symbol to relate the central integrity of his self to ethnic identity. Although reared as a Jew, he never felt Jewish, but like an impostor. In an effort to make his life more Jewish, he married a Jewish girl and became an anthropologist specializing in life in early Israel.

In this case, as in all others we analyzed, the fabric of mental life was woven from many threads, from Freudian to ethnic, and it is not surprising that when neurosis develops, we are dealing with a tangled skein. Value judgments are always implied—and often explicit—in feelings of ethnic identity, so feelings of personal worth and worthlessness are often played out in the ethnic area. Some of the criteria for judgments have intensely personal and idiosyncratic qualities, but many have the universal qualities Pinderhughes (1982) writes about, as evidenced by two simple but dramatic examples that occurred in a single family.

Vignette 4

Two sisters who grew up in an Italian-American family reacted very differently to conflicts related to ethnic issues. As in so many of our cases, the ethnic issues were intertwined with issues of sexual identity and pregenital conflicts.

The maternal side of the family was northern Italian and of fair complexion, the paternal, Sicilian and dark. Family values and attitudes reinforced the association of southern with what was dark, impulsive, dirty, and sexual. Whereas the fair-skinned sister was sexually inhibited, the younger brunette was sexually promiscuous, often with black men. Both sought treatment. That of the younger, whose expressiveness facilitated therapeutic intervention, progressed more rapidly; the older sister's inhibitions were linked to a character structure that was modified only very slowly in analytic treatment.

One need not be a student of family dynamics to appreciate that a case of this sort represents another instance of role assignment in family life. The conscious or unconscious parental choice of one child to be the good child and another to be the bad is often determined by factors of the Pinderhughes and ethnic types, and we see this phenomenon widespread at the social level too. It is also of diverse kinds, from the selection of criminals to the selection of leaders (we will return to the latter subject shortly). By analogy to what Freud called "neuroses of destiny," society's victims and elect have lives of destiny.

Incest and exogamy, the taboos that govern sexuality and reproduction, have long interested behavioral scientists of various disciplines. In the next case vignette we focus on the interplay of reality and fantasy in the sets of mental representations that contribute to object relations. Although this case resulted in a clinical neurosis, the underlying dynamics are universal. They include the dynamics of stereotype formation from familial and societal indoctrination, blended with fragments of real or fantasied "actual experience." On analysis, it can be seen that the latter comprises much that is externalized and projected, indicating a form of construction toward the object, to borrow a term from perceptgenesis.

Vignette 5

Our next case is that of a woman of Greek Orthodox background who married a Jewish professor during the time when her mother lay dying. Her husband made it clear in advance that he wanted his children to be reared as Jews. He was very happily attached to his parental family, in poignant contrast to his wife's sadness over her mother's terminal illness. Her distress was all the worse for having a background of unresolved oedipal attachment to and reaction against her father, a man who had no doubt that everything Greek was good and everything foreign, bad. But she agreed to her husband's condition, hoping that he would be able to make their new family the center of his life, which she strove to do despite her grief.

For some years she was disturbed by her husband's attachment to his family, but tolerated it. When she became pregnant, her conflict intensified even though he tried to help. When ultrasound revealed that the child was a boy, her conflict became unbearable as she imagined herself bearing and rearing "a Jewish boy." She sought psychotherapy; this focused on sorting out the transfer of attachments and conflicts from her family of origin to her new family—a problem she had recognized in her husband but now came to acknowledge in herself.

Of particular interest was that the patient in imagining herself rearing "a Jewish boy" was haunted by images of the one Jewish boy she had known in her childhood. Her profound dislike for him had centered on personality traits that in her personal family and ethnic experience had been disowned and attributed to others. Some of these personal traits were characterized as Jewish by her culture and family, so it was more readily possible for her to deny these in herself and find them in her young Jewish neighbor. This case is a graphic illustration of the way the reciprocal power of personal and social dynamics contributes to the momentum of stereotyping.

Interracial and mixed marriages often represent (at least in part) successful attempts to escape and transcend what some individuals have felt to be the constrictions of race and religion. Despite sincere repudiation of prejudice, some elements of hatred and its vicissitudes (e. g., externalization, projection, and denial) may remain embedded in the personality structure and reassert themselves in later times of personal trial.

The person with a bicultural background occupies what is virtually by definition an ambiguous position. Although he enjoys being able to relate to both camps as "the man at the margin," he is vulnerable to identity diffusion with all of its discomforts. When psychiatric illness strikes such an individual, it is not unusual to see issues of personal identity elaborated in ethnic terms.

Vignette 6

Bob Kafumi (pseudonym), a 31-year-old West African, came to the United States to enter an undergraduate program in electrical engineering at a major university. He had been an honor student in Africa, but he was socially unadventurous and highly dependent on his mother. In his eighteenth year he replaced his African name with the name *Bob* in preparation for coming to America. Although descended from high tribal officials, including medicine men, his family had become Christians a generation earlier.

During his undergraduate years in Boston he met and married an East African woman 10 years his senior. They had three children. While his wife was pregnant with their first child, several months after Bob graduated from college, he suffered the first of several psychotic episodes and was hospitalized with a diagnosis of manic-depressive illness. His mental condition cleared within a few weeks, and he was able to resume his previous high level of functioning in a technical job. He also began psychotherapy, addressing concerns about his ability to advance from his role as student to function effectively as a man and head of a family.

During this time ambiguous circumstances about his wife's background came to light. He was surprised to learn that before coming to America she had borne a son, now 14, by a soldier who had been killed during political turmoil. She had left her son to be cared for in Africa by her brother's family, but the boy's uncle decided to terminate the arrangement because of political pressures and family stress. It was decided that the teenager would join his mother and live with her new family in the United States.

At this point, two years after terminating his first course of psychotherapy, Bob reentered therapy to seek help in coping with this major event. After the teenager arrived, the resulting tensions in the family proved too much for Bob. He again became psychotic, with mixed bipolar symptoms, aggressive behavioral changes, accusatory auditory hallucinations, and an inability to function effectively as a professional and as a father. He was hospitalized. During this psychotic episode he rejected his Christian name and insisted on being addressed by his African one, saying that this was who he really was. At this point he confronted fears that he would not be able to work at the level of his education in a high tech position since he felt weak and ineffectual. He defended against these fears by using his African name and proudly affirming his identity as an African from an important family, but he also continued reading the Bible as an additional source of strength during this difficult period. When the psychotic episode abated, he again referred to himself as Bob. His treatment focused on integrating sources of self-esteem from his ethnic heritage in Africa and his academic achievements in the West. He made good improvement and was able to obtain a professional job as a project engineer.

Psychological well-being is heavily dependent on a state of harmony and contact amounting to continuity with the environment, human and nonhuman. Such continuity is for the most part taken for granted, underestimated, or even denied. Western cultures value individuality and independence and nurture an ego ideal that assumes the ability always to "go it alone." We are taught early to reject and deny the loneliness and homesickness of leaving what is comfortably familiar.

In certain circumstances intense continuity with others has favorable social sanction or at least some toleration. The inseparability of lovers and of mother and infant is well respected, probably because of its necessity for the survival of the species. But for the greater part of adult life, the assumption is that the person is sufficient unto himself and does not need others to serve as parts of himself and to make him whole. A similar need for a familiar and fairly constant physical and cultural environment to serve as self objects and assure the integrity of the individual is seldom consciously appreciated.

Travel away from familiar people and familiar culture usually proves to be a pleasant and stimulating challenge to the personality. But if the challenging circumstances are too intense and the personality is in a vulnerable state, travel or relocation may result in psychological disorganization (Barnes 1980). We now present a case vignette that illustrates how psychological homeostasis is imperiled by the lack of familiar people, culture, and places.

Vignette 7

A middle-aged, well-adjusted Indian scientist who had never traveled abroad was appointed to the faculty of an American university. He was to precede his family to the United States by a few months, and recognizing his vulnerability to loneliness, he got the names and addresses of fellow Indians he might contact in America. His foreboding was well founded; he was lonely and homesick from the start and thought constantly of his wife, children, and grandchildren, and of India. He wept a great deal, lost his concentration, and was unable to work. An empty, drained, and anergic feeling haunted him. Anorexia, insomnia, and vague physical complaints developed; a major depression ensued.

His struggle against loneliness and depression drew heavily on ethnic themes and illustrates the need of self-objects. He was miserable alone in his apartment and complained that it was "useless to look out the window as there was no one in the street." "In India," he explained, "you can't look anywhere without seeing people!" He sought Indian food but found it difficult to get what he wanted since he was a strict vegetarian. He wandered the city streets until late at night just to see people, but he felt unable to talk to any of those he saw. He called one of his Indian contacts and asked him to come and stay with him at night. But his contact was "too Americanized and too busy to be any help," and although the patient went to stay with this contact, he soon left for the house of another Indian, where he found a little relief since that family was more Indian. He continued to be obsessed with India and those he knew and cared for there. At night he had many dreams, mostly about people and the joy of finding those he knew, being reunited with them, and once again speaking in his native tongue. In desperation he phoned his wife and pleaded with her and the children to "come and save" him.

Vignette 8

One final case illustrates the defensive use of a strong nationalistic identification, one in which an exaggerated sense of belonging in a majority culture was used by a member of a minority group to defend against troubling emotions and conflict within the primary family unit. This defensive configuration resulted chiefly from a family tragedy that obscured, or diverted, this man's development and caused emotional arrests and the elaboration of defensive structures that relied partly on this nationalistic identification.

Martin, a successful professional man from an eastern European country, sought psychoanalysis at the age of 37 because of "depression." In the capital city of his youth, Martin's parents and extended family isolated themselves within the Jewish community, and stayed away from the majority cultural and religious group. As a teenager Martin did the opposite and formed an intense attachment to a non-Jewish peer group. The relationships he formed in this group gave him the strongest feeling of belonging he had ever had.

He was the adored, first of three children in the family of a successful Jewish merchant. When he was five, a baby brother was born. Martin seems to have adapted well to this event, but when the baby was 14 months old and Martin just over six, the baby, with whom Martin had enjoyed playing, fell ill and was given the wrong medication by their father. Martin recalled that a doctor gave the weak and bloated infant some injections, but the baby failed rapidly and died, evidently as a result of the father's mistake.

The family was plunged into deep mourning. The father, who had given the child what was thought to be the lethal agent, was consumed by grief and guilt. From Martin's point of view, as it was reconstructed during his analysis, there seemed no way to relieve his parents of their desolation and guilt, which he felt was his responsibility. He remembered asking his father, "Am I not enough?"

A sister's birth, less than a year after the baby's death, further damaged Martin's special position within the family. As time went by, Judaism, with its emphasis on guilt and the victimization of the Jewish people, became psychologically linked with the family tragedy. The atmosphere of "doom and gloom" and anxiety about survival that dominated his family and his parents' relationship to him was connected in his mind with a somber, joyless view of Judaism and the Jewish experience. In his midteens Martin became greatly attached to the non-Jewish peer group, which enjoyed picnics, sports, and sexual exploration together. Martin idealized everything about his native city that was not Jewish—its buildings, cuisine, and smells, its view of the harbor, and even its crowds.

Martin came to the United States at 18 to enlarge his intellectual gifts and pursue professional opportunities. When he was married and the father of a one-year-old daughter, the unresolved conflicts of his childhood drove him to seek treatment. It soon became evident that although he had lived half his life in the United States, he had never felt that he belonged there. His emotional identification remained almost altogether with the peer group in his homeland, which he continued to idealize in spite of being aware of the terrible economic and political problems they faced.

His longings and dreams centered on images and scenes of his native city and country and, above all, on memories of the enjoyable summers spent with his adolescent group. He felt like a displaced, isolated person in the United States, although he was hard working and highly successful in his profession. He fantasied returning some day to his native land, being welcomed as a hero, and being put in charge of one of the ministries related to his field.

After two years in analysis he told a story his father had told him when he was a child; it captured the quality of his developmental arrest:

> A fairy godmother gave a five-year-old boy a magic bobbin. This bobbin allowed the child to have wishes that would come true but that could not be undone. All the child had to do was to pull out the thread. First, he wished he could be seven, to have more privileges; then, when he was seven, he wished he

could be twelve to enjoy the rights and privileges of a twelve-year-old. And so it went, until he was an old man and there was very little thread left. Then, realizing that he had not really lived at all, he wanted to wind the thread back, but the fairy godmother said, "No, you cannot go back, for the thread winds in only one direction."

Through this tale Martin saw that his whole life had been so governed by childhood fantasies and imaginings, that he had not been able to take much pleasure in his ongoing life. As he looked more deeply into his psychological fixations, he discovered the many ways in which the period surrounding the death of his baby brother had produced intolerable conflicts for him within the family. Although he had realized at the time that a tragedy had occurred, he could not deal with or understand his parents' withdrawal into their preoccupation with the loss of their infant. Martin's efforts to compensate for this loss through his own "good works," especially his achievements at school, were all to no avail.

His identification with his Jewish origins, the ethnic identification that dominated the life of his family, became associated with intolerable pain and loss. He devalued his parents, who seemed joyless and caught up in depression and anxiety. Understandably, after the baby's death they had become oversolicitous and anxious about Martin's well-being, panicking at the slightest indication that he might be unhappy or that something might be wrong and being unable to appreciate accomplishments that were important to him. This pattern had continued into his adult life, and ultimately he rejected the experience of love and family belongingness. As boys in latency and adolescence tend to do, Martin turned to his peer group for friendship and for the expansion of his capacity for relationships, but his identification with the group was exaggerated, greatly idealized, and maintained at the expense of relationships within the family.

His case illustrates the way in which an exaggerated nationalistic identification can be used to avoid affects and conflicts originating within the nuclear family. In turn, as in this case, nationalistic identification can also prevent healthy progress in the capacity to belong appropriately to new adult groups, organizations, and societies.

It is important to explore the defensive as well as the primary functions of ethnic and nationalistic identification, as in any other group identifications. Membership in a national group can provide a strong sense of belonging and a positive self-esteem for an individual who has a number of healthy group identifications, but it may also represent a more primitive defensive strategy that serves to avoid the affects and hurts associated with conflicted early attachments within the family, particularly those related to unresolved grief, mourning, and loss.

The Leader and the Group

The relationship between leader and group is a focal factor in the expression of both current and historical ethnicity. It is central in the achievement of present ethnonational political goals and crucial for a people seeking new solutions in situations of crisis.

This relationship has been studied from many points of view; here we shall speak mainly of its "object relations" aspects. Each of the partners—the group and its leader—treats the other, both consciously and unconsciously, as an object that represents significant elements of past life and the expected future. For each partner the other constitutes, symbolically and sometimes concretely, an extension of his own life; each uses the other, and each creates the other.

Karl Marx believed that every social era needs its own great personages and if there is no such personage, it will create one. And Freud (1933/1964) spoke of the necessary dyad of followers and leaders, writing in an uncharacteristically categorical way to Einstein that "One instance of the innate and ineradicable inequality of men is their tendency to fall into the two classes of leaders and followers" (p. 212). He then continued his absolutism, though softening it a little: "The latter constitute the vast majority; they

stand in need of an authority which will make decisions for them
and to which they for the most part offer an unqualified submis-
sion" (p. 212).

Weber (1967) notes that charismatic leaders come to power in
times of crisis. A certain "fit" or congruity between the leader and
his followers is vital (Volkan & Itzkowitz, 1984). A true charismatic
leader must possess a constellation of conscious and unconscious
personal psychodynamics that correspond to the group's needs,
and in turn he must be able to satisfy his own psychological needs
in dealing with his group. The way he heals the reduced self-
esteem of a people struggling with seemingly unsurmountable
problems depends on his personality organization and how it fits
with societal conditions. Hitler strengthened German self-confidence
by degrading and brutalizing others as pseudospecies, but other
leaders have healed group injury by rallying the people around
traditional national images. Churchill did this constructively and
creatively; Khomeini does it by regressive hate-filled appeals to
fundamentalism.

Although there are fixed and even stereotyped aspects of the
leader/follower relationship, there is also something continually
changing and dynamic about it. Although all truly transforming
leaders are charismatic and appear only at a time of crisis and
disorganization as a focus for reorganization, the changes they
bring about may in fact bring radically altered ethnicity or an
altered national purpose. Quite uncharismatic and indeed rather
ordinary leaders are indispensable in promoting the assimilation
of change and the maintenance of the new or updated ethnic
identity. A charismatic leader may need a number of such "assimilators"
to help the group integrate a new set of mental representations into
its self-concept.

Crisis not only stirs feelings of ethnonationalism, it intensifies
the group/leader relationship; ethnonationalism readily becomes
the medium of exchange in this trade, enhancing the self-esteem
of each member of the dyad. The greater the danger, the greater
the need to raise self-esteem; increased self-esteem powers political action. The messianic or charismatic leader is apt to have a

sense of self or egotism that approaches or reaches the grandiose, although he may take pains to appear humble; the dynamics of both leader and group freely utilize this grandiosity. The leader's psychological impact depends on a kind of continuous updating of reciprocal interaction rather than on the person of the leader alone. But the way he handles this dynamic is largely determined by his own psychological makeup. Volkan (1981) has identified two types of charismatic, narcissistic leadership: the reparative and the destructive.

Reparative Leadership

The reparative leader tries to raise the status of his people in order to win the love of what is thereby recognized as a superior race. His efforts may then foster among them a new sense of ethnonationality.

In a psychobiographical study of Atatürk, Volkan and Itzkowitz (1984) illuminate the remarkable fit between the makeup of Atatürk and the critical need of his native Turkey. At the time of Atatürk's ascendancy his country was suffering from a protracted war that had cost many casualties and the loss of territory and prestige. Born into a house of mourning to a grief-stricken mother, Atatürk as a small child felt an unconscious mission to "repair" his mother. He found his chance to carry out this mission in a displaced way by healing the grieving Turkish nation. For reasons that combined his own personal object-relations needs and Turkey's need to modernize, he led his people to a new sense of identity.

Volkan (1972, 1979) also tells of the touching solution a people found when political circumstances prevented the emergence of a leader. In Cyprus between 1963 and 1968, the Turks, numerically a minority on the island, were forced by island Greeks into ghettoes surrounded by U.N. peacekeeping forces with Greek troops at their outer circumference. For five years Cypriot Turks were virtual prisoners within their enclaves, where physical conditions were very poor. Their shared hardship strengthened their sense of ethnicity; their erstwhile leaders were in exile or rendered helpless, and in their subjugated state they could not create one, so they expressed their need for a leader or saviour in a curious and complex way by raising thousands of parakeets in cages. The birds were everywhere, in homes, coffee shops, and grocery stores.

The Turks lived in congested quarters with large extended families and mirrored their situation by keeping several birds in each cage. The link between the condition of the birds and that of the people was further illustrated by the comical practice of identifying biologically unrelated birds as father, mother, grandfather, and so on. While the caged birds represented the mass of needy and victimized Turks, they also gave the latter the opportunity to act as saviours. The Turks took care of their birds, making sure they were well fed and happy. Thus, in the absence of a leader they dramatized their need and to some degree assuaged it.

Destructive Leadership

The charismatic leader functioning in a destructive, narcissistic way has his followers join him in devaluing the other group, raising their self-esteem as well as his own by comparison with the devalued group. He may emphasize the established ethnic identity, or create a new one, but the process is unstable and potentially dangerous as ethnicity is being enhanced by reducing the other group's self-esteem; differences are emphasized, boundaries strengthened, and any likeness to the opposing group denied. This makes each group regard the other as a despised subspecies whose existence justifies destructive aggression.

Terrorists and terrorism would appear to be the total antithesis of group-approved leaders and such state-approved violence as certain police actions and war. But they have their origins in the same group systems of object relations, mental representations, and personifications.

Terrorism on the part of a segment of a community is a painful challenge to the whole community and especially to its leaders. Moral revulsion at the violence of terrorism is usually widely shared and expressed by political leaders. Ultranationalism is often blamed and it is pointed out that the organization involved, the IRA, Gush Emunim, or the like, is supported by only a small minority of the people. The denial is too often scapegoating or, at worst, hypocritical. It is forgotten for the moment that the community has helped to generate through quite respectable educational means the ethnic, religious, and nationalistic spirit that underlies the actions.

Fanatical terrorists are often pitiful and pitiless people who have grown up in an either/or environment; they have no tolerance for ambiguity, and therefore no tolerance for others. A rigid, grandiose identification with idealized images of national heroes and myths enables the terrorist to assume the task of what he thinks is national salvation. He becomes the personification and, if we may use a violent metaphor, the spearhead of the national spirit as it has too often been taught to him in the unambiguous and simplistic terms of national myth and history. Terrorists really feel they are heroes and that they are right, and soon the timid majority will join and acclaim them. And sometimes they are right, at least in that their nationalism works. It did for quite a while for the Nazis.

When hit by the dreadful force of a terrorist act, it is comforting for the community to think of ambivalence (if they think of it at all) as being, like differing political positions, divided among different population groups. We are speaking here of the tendency to ascribe differing opinions and feelings about the act to different groups in the population. In fact these opinions and feelings are not so neatly compartmentalized but are widely shared. Sincere soul-searching, which is often possible only when removed from the occasion, will reveal the secret condoning or even approval by the majority of the acts they themselves condemn. In saying that such ambivalence is universal, we allow that it is of differing intensity from person to person.

Terrorism, then, is an opportunity for the simplistic politician and churchman. The righteous are bold and there is quick comfort in strident condemnation of the villains. A favored adjective in describing terrorists' actions is "cowardly," an oddly provocative way of describing men who give their lives in suicide bombings and starve themselves to death. They might well ask, "If this is cowardice how can we show courage?" The usual consequence of this taunting is further escalation of the violence.

Terrorism can't be condoned but neither should it be enhanced by mindless provocative rhetoric. The fanatic is thus driven to further degrees of merger with his ideology and group, which induces an omnipotent disdain for his immediate personal mortality in favor of grandiose notions of immortality as the hero, and at a still deeper level, as the people itself. Among the many measures needed to cope with terrorism is leadership that recognizes the psychological complicity of the community in supporting extremism. It is rare indeed to find a churchman or politician who questions his people's way of indoctrinating the young with highly idealized representations of national heroes, exaggerations of wrongs inflicted on the nation, and distorted images of the "enemy."

Leaders, whether group sanctioned, revolutionaries, or terrorists, are the symbols and realizations of a group's system of object relationships. Such systems and leaders in some degree represent sets of frozen attitudes and ways of relating to the world based on a people's history and pseudohistory. Trapped in such views and behavior that have the quality of a collective "repetition-compulsion," leaders and groups too often are unable to relate to other groups and occasions as they actually are. We turn in the next chapter to some of the intra- and intergroup vicissitudes of these processes.

5
ETHNICITY IN GROUP AND INTERGROUP RELATIONS

This chapter makes some observations concerning large group and intergroup behavior in the light of object relations theory, previously introduced. One historical impetus for this study of ethnonationalism was the resurgence in the United States during the late 1960s and 1970s of what is often called the New Ethnicity. Whether exemplified in the Afro-American movement, the Native American movement, and so on, a resurgence of interest in ethnic identity has paralleled the fragmentation of the American dream in the aftermath of the assassinations of those idealized leaders, John and Robert Kennedy and Martin Luther King, Jr. The ensuing national mourning process can be viewed as an attempt to *restore* a sense of lost identity by searching for roots. In a series of papers (Stein, 1975a, 1979; Stein & Hill, 1977b) and in the book *The Imperative: Examining the New White Ethnic Movement* (Stein & Hill, 1977a), Stein explored the history and shared psychological aspects of this process. Ethnicity is shown in this monograph to serve the function of relieving anxiety when prior group identifications have failed.

We emphasize again that a group tends to become preoccupied with the integrity of its identity and political boundaries in times of crisis, rigidly defining what and who is to be included, and what excluded (if not expelled). Thus the Black Power movement polarized blacks and whites; and the white ethnics, such as Irish, Polish, Slovaks, and Italians, radically differentiated themselves from blacks and from those they disparaged as predominantly white Anglo-Saxon Protestants (WASPs). These newly distinguished "ethnicities" must on no account be mistaken for the erstwhile cultures of origin from which their participants claim descent. Stein and Hill (1977a) distinguish between a "behavioral ethnicity," which members take unselfconsciously for granted and "ideological ethnicity," a polemical, evaluative assertion and quest for what can no longer be taken for granted. It is the psychological use and meaning of culture rather than the fact or specific content of a culture per se that occupies our attention here.

Since the late 1970s up to the present time (1987) there has been an interesting resurgence of what can be called American ethno-nationalism; this has strongly emerged without apparent contradiction from the many who have loudly asserted their pride in their ancestral culture and disdain for anything "WASP." This new sense of American identity is symbolized if not personified in President Ronald Reagan, in whom "ethnic" and "nationalist" aspirations meet. In the 1960s and 1970s interest in many of the constituent ethnicities of the United States was revitalized as investment in the American dream declined. We see today, however, a symbolic "linking" or condensation of ethnic sentiments with American national sentiments and ambitions, all consolidated in the group representation of President Reagan, who promises the restoration of American pride, purpose, and wholeness. Many Americans, irrespective of ethnic ancestry, currently identify their primary group affiliation as American. Just as the New Ethnicity earlier gained internal cohesion by opposing the American culture, today's revitalized American nationalistic identity is unified in renewed strenuous opposition to the nearest thing America has to a perceived common historic enemy, Communist Russia. This current process of mutual identification of ethnic group members as primarily Americans with emergent popular leaders is an example of the dynamics of burgeoning collective identities worldwide. For an earlier example the reader is referred to Kohn's (1960) seminal work on *Pan-Slavism*, which tells of people gathering under a new and wider umbrella of collectivity, or *"Pan-ism,"* for protection from the pain of identity wounded by history's outrageous misfortunes.

In this chapter we explore the potential vicissitudes of object relations in group aspects of ethnicity. The distinction between intragroup and intergroup process is moot, because what is perceived as taking place outside the group is not only essential to but, paradoxically, part of what takes place within it. Both group processes are aspects of the same phenomenon: a social identity at once self- and object-oriented. That is, an ethnic group identity may be built on such riddance mechanisms as externalization, projection, and projective identification, in which the inner-core group identity is sustained, while at the same time the ethnic group remains bound to devalued nongroup members.

It is often argued that group membership and group identity are adaptive. We should explain our use of the term *adaptation* in connection with ethnicity. To refer to some human behavior as adaptive is usually to locate it as meaningful and promoting sur- vival with reference to a particular human *Umwelt* or social ecology— for example, a family, an ethnic group, or a nation. Moreover, to label some human behavior as adaptive is often to indicate tacit approval. However, these are decidedly *not* the way this term is used here.

Ours is a biological orientation; here the adaptive or maladap- tive "unit" must be the species—which refuses to perceive itself as a single species. Ethnicity is homeostatic when experienced from within the group; each group uses intergroup instability as a defense mechanism to promote intragroup stability. Contamination of the outer environment serves to ensure and promote the purity of the inner environment. Ethnicity thus reveals a paradox in adaptation; on the one hand, it fosters the group's survival and cohesion, but on the other hand, it may in the long run endanger its future. By splitting off and allocating group-dystonic attributes to others, a group may limit its alternatives and therefore its adaptability. It is both paradox and irony that self-protection may unwittingly con- tribute to self-destruction.

In terms of the costs and consequences to the group, ethnicity can be seen as potentially maladaptive in its quest for that perfect homeostasis between the good-inside and the bad-outside. Not only do preservation and jeopardy of the precious group inner environment go hand-in-hand, but ethnicity depends likewise on the reduction of reality testing (which, after all, is the final arbiter

of adaptation) and intergenerational transmission of that reduction. One cannot truly know a devalued adversary or an idealized
ally realistically when that enemy or friend must serve as a repository of parts of one's own group.

To survive individually and as a species we must relinquish the
very aspect of ethnic exclusivity that we have used to accomplish
countless unconscious tasks. We must be willing to attempt to
examine unconscious process in group behaviors. Consider, for
instance, the hypothesized oedipal and counteroedipal functions
of interethnic and international warfare. The hypotheses involved
are, of course, quite controversial and doubtless not always dominant or even highly contributory as causes of war. One does not
have to endorse them to recognize that the system in which they
may play a part is now made vulnerable by nuclear weapons.

In the past, fathers sent sons to battle to die for the father and
motherland; sons could kill other rivalrous sons and perhaps lay
waste to concretely symbolized mother and fatherlands, victoriously
conquering and claiming other men's motherlands, making restitution for their oedipal guilt by suffering or dying for their father
and motherlands (see Walsh & Scandalis, 1975). With the threat of
nuclear war, fathers have now lost the opportunity to kill their sons
and survive the filicide. In the past one could kill the enemy
without losing one's own life, but this is no longer possible. Oedipal
jeopardy in turn jeopardizes the father. Oedipal and counteroedipal
aggression become fused: to kill one's son, one's enemies' sons, and
fathers is to commit suicide. Similarly, the sadism and masochism
that could be, if only tenuously, split in earlier wars are now fused:
to kill is to be killed. To survive now we have literally no choice but
to examine and foreswear the impulse to act out oedipal and
counteroedipal rivalries. The pseudotherapy of inflicting pain on
an adversary must make way for the far more difficult liberating
pain of learning to tolerate, understand, and comprehend the
timeless strife between fathers and sons.

If we answer the question "What are groups *for?*" with the reply
"survival," we take into account only external environmental conditions and overlook the issues of psychic survival. Group bounda-

ries exist to give cohesiveness to the group-self; to exclude its disavowed parts; to prevent fusion with others; and to keep disowned parts of the group-self at a safe distance, embodied by one's enemies. Groups usually cling to a sense of their own collective goodness, but some identify totally and vehemently with a "negative identity" (Erikson, 1968), renouncing the good one to embrace a bad one that self-consciously violates its predecessor.

The terms "good" and "bad" are used somewhat uniquely in a psychoanalytic context, referring respectively to bipolar pleasurable and unpleasurable (painful) self- and object representations. Good affective representational units tend to be invested with libido; bad ones with aggression. Although these terms are intended to be developmentally descriptive rather than moralistic, their retention in psychoanalytic writing attests to their unconscious appropriateness in analytic vocabulary. Also, the early splits they indicate lie at the heart of primitive superego development and its profound either/or moralisms. Later applications owe something to early patterned experiences and internalized structures. Valuing the integration (mending) of opposing affectively tinged self- and object representations as a sign of greater maturity than splitting, we may conclude that being preoccupied with "goodness" and "badness" promotes violence even as we seek the good.

There are still groups in the world whose propensity to violence is ego-syntonic and considerably higher and more recurrent than is usual in the West. This statement may seem an ethnocentric slur, but this is not our intention. We simply indicate that although all groups have an integrative potential or capacity, different ones have attained different levels of that integration, and higher levels give way to more primitive ones when regression occurs. It marks an evolutionary advance for wanton violence and destruction to become ego-dystonic to a group, and unacceptable rather than unconsciously gratifying.

Structural anthropologists attempting to account for ethnic persistence tend to refer to Levi-Strauss (1963), Barth (1969), and Leach (1964) and to argue that "While cultural distinctiveness may be a necessary condition for an ethnic identity . . . for ethnic boundaries to persist there must be structural opposition between groups" (Hamilton, 1981, p. 953). By omitting issues at the level of self and affect, they miss what the opposition is about and stress economic competition and bipolar cognitive classifications based on alleged brain structure.

Ethnicity well illustrates the role of projection in the regulation of group identity and intergroup relations and perceptions. It can be viewed as a *projectively constituted social system beyond and successor to the family;* the bad is expelled outside the system's boundary so the good may be retained within it. Goodness that members of the group feel unattainable in the group itself is found in out-groups, with which the groups feels in some way affiliated.

Ethnicity is alternately experienced as a maternal object one depends on and a predifferentiated, symbiotic self-object. Since stress threatens homeostasis and we use ethnicity to restabilize the group, it is no wonder that we defend our bands, tribes, chiefdoms, ethnic groups, and nation-states with such unchecked vehemence. And no wonder our ethnocentrisms often become rigid. For each people, whatever the social scale or level of complexity, is the symbolic heir to imperfect mother-child unions that we fantasize in the present as having been perfect.

One could argue that what many contemporary writers discuss under the term *ethnicity,* is one among several cultic-regressive responses to the disappointments and disillusionments of the culture. When a culture inevitably fails to meet human need, its members renew, revitalize, and refashion their culture to restore what has been lost. The more regressive the group dynamics, the more defensive ethnicity becomes. In the United States the "New Ethnicity" is such a cult in the symbolism of the nation-state.

This perspective on the unconscious precursors symbolized in ethnicity requires reexamination of what we think we know about ethnicity. Levi-Strauss (1967), as a structural anthropologist, notes that intergroup perceptions and relations are often governed by a principle of binary opposition. Likewise, Barth (1969), one of the leading theoreticians of "ethnic groups and boundaries," advances a model of group complementarity based on 1) contrasting intergroup values and other cultural characteristics, and 2) rules of interaction that preserve the integrity of boundaries. Each participant member is thus able to maintain his or her separate distinct identity both despite and because members may cross one another's boundaries for mutually advantageous business transactions. What these models do not account for is the persistent *need* for the opposition, insistence on distinctness, and vigilant border patrol.

A culture's language evokes we/they distinctions in the service of what Spicer (1971) calls the principle of opposition. Vocabulary, accents, names, and communicating gestures; moral differences; political activities; land; music and art; folk heroes, and so on all become enlisted as boundary-setting symbols, their function being to clearly include (what is "good") and exclude (what is "bad") so there will be no question as to who and what belongs where.

"Insiders" (those who identify themselves and/or who are identified as belonging together) and "outsiders" (those defined and/or who define themselves as not belonging—foreigners) develop markers that define the boundaries and thereby become a social group's cultural symbols. They are interesting for their cultural content within a group (e.g., language, religion, and dress), but we must not lose sight of the intergroup context that gives the content its significance. One's whoness and the other's otherness are constantly being defined and negotiated, both within and without the group, in the form of reciprocal projection and introjection. Any content can be conscripted into the service of boundary delineation, as we see in the following vignettes.

Vignette 1

Early in this century one focus of conflict in America between Catholics of the Latin rite and those of the Byzantine was whether it was proper to carry pussywillow or palm branches in church on Palm Sunday. The Byzantine custom in east-central Europe favored the former. Also, Byzantine Catholics crossed themselves from right to left, but Latin rite Catholics did so from left to right. These apparently small differences in ritual, already divisive in Europe, were highly significant in America. These differences were used for the purposes of differentiation on the part of Byzantine rite Catholics, and assimilation-acculturation pressure on the part of Latin rite Catholics. What began as an historic religious conflict was absorbed into a later ethnonationalist conflict between Rusyns and Slovaks (for instance), as religion became part of the content of ethnonationalist conflict. In studying this process one must not be overly fascinated with the content of the difference but should examine the context of the often desperate need to create boundaries that serve the purpose of differentiation.

Vignette 2

This example illustrates how cultural material is exploited in choosing a name to symbolically resolve an identity difficulty. While attending a conference, an Israeli-born Jewish-American in his thirties commented at length on a paper that dealt with the psychological significance of Jewish names and name changes. Although he had originally used the diaspora name his parents had given him, he had, after much soul-searching, changed it to a Hebrew-Israeli one that translated into English his original first name, plus a patronymic. He explained that he had perceived his father as a weak, ineffectual, traditional diaspora Jew, and he wanted an identity of his own. He spoke of the profound importance of one's name in self-identity and recalled the biblical story involving symbolic struggles over one's name and, by extension, the name of the group with which one affiliated and from which one claimed descent and inheritance.

This conflict and its tenuous solution(s) are hardly idiosyncratic but lie at the heart of the Zionist movement, the ideology of the Sabra (Israeli native), and the relationship between Israel and diaspora Jewry (see Gonen, 1975). The Israeli nationalist identity repudiated the diaspora past and had to contend with the past through the future. Moreover, precisely because what is at issue is the meaning of cultural material, we should note how cultural symbols and ideology express personal and familial conflicts through externalization. Recall how many American blacks renounced their slave names during the late 1960s and the 1970s, adopting African or Arabic ones. This suggests that not only is social role internalized, but also personal and group identity depends on externalizations that complement what has been internalized.

The greater the sense of internal or external threat, the more necessary it is that boundaries to be closed and anything threatening inner perfection be excluded by linguistic, cultural, and demographic purging (Czigany, 1974). Geographical boundaries take on psychological meanings. Old primitive meanings are brought into play as though a homeland were mother and the adversary, the oedipal father. Metaphor is concretized as the regressed self voraciously expands its boundaries to encompass everything possible. Appetite becomes insatiable; adults now see the world as they did when infants who thought themselves omnipotent in spite of their real condition of vulnerability. The early border conflicts over differentiating the self from the other are now being addressed by an infant in the body of an adult, one whose efforts to implement his/her most primitive fantasies unleash unbridled idealization and brutality. Infantile disputes over the borders within the family are displaced and projected onto the stage of society.

The frightened nationalist must renegotiate some of the most crucial developmental issues: Where do I begin and end? How can I keep myself together? How can I avert engulfment-annihilation or disappearance-annihilation? But as an adult one feels an insatiable need for more than simple survival and views one's ambitions as invincible and one's resources as infinite. Although one feels entitled to the realization of one's dreams, one is much threatened by annihilation, separation, loss, abandonment, and castration. Expansionism is a reaction to the fear of loss. It is idle to ask, in terms of demographic reality, "How much land is enough?" without taking into account what land means symbolically to those demanding even more of it.

Nationalists use self- and other-representations, speaking of blood ties, descent, origin, siblinghood and the like, not in a chiefly political reference, but because they are now organizing their inner world according to those early experiences and relationships that had offered the most security.

In the Pan-Slavism of the late 19th century many of the lesser Slavic peoples saw themselves as the younger brothers of Russia, that gigantic and powerful older brother to the east and north (Kohn, 1960). In the 1960s and 1970s many U.S. citizens whose original homeland or ancestry lay in Slavic east-central Europe began to regard themselves as threatened by those whom they disparagingly called WASPs. Many Slovak-, Polish-, Croatian-, and other Slavic-Americans began to see themselves as disregarded if not abused junior siblings and WASPs as sinister, rejecting older siblings and parents. Likewise, American black nationalists began calling each other "Brother" and "Sister" about the same time (Stein, 1979; Stein & Hill, 1973, 1977a).

Family metaphor is common in ethnonationalist rhetoric, sentiment, and ideology. Its unconscious mythology serves the chief function of stabilizing the group when personal identity is confused. Kafka and McDonald (1965) describe that in families having fluid boundaries among members, the sense of "subjective equivalence" among various family members confers a sense of corporate continuity when the sense of individuality has dissolved. In ethnonationalist groups and movements the fantasy and mythology of the familial character of the group performs the same psychological function. This borrowed and shared fictive-sibling kinship identity patches up defective personal identity structures and helps to stabilize both the internal and group environment.

When regressed, erstwhile strangers not only relate closely but also feel united by a sense of fate and common identity, each merging indistinguishably into the other, all becoming members of one mythical family. Progressive dedifferentiation occurs within the newly constituted group, and discrimination against the out-group becomes more and more exacting.

There are disappointments in the group symbiosis, however; it is not perfect, but needs constant repair, being fraught also with the danger of engulfment and annihilation. It is a tricky psychic maneuver to be at one with the group but not consumed by it; ethnic symbiosis has a certain tentative quality and some, though not all, functions regress. Such regression is never altogether an expression of id impulses but is always object-related also, designed to repair old wounds, to return to old conflicts to try mastering them once and for all. But such final and complete resolution is not forthcoming, and solutions often put additional burdens on the group.

A recurrent, if not constant, theme in the history of nationalist movements is the *expansion of identity boundaries.* The transference of the individual's narcissistic and voracious needs and terrors onto the group is not limited to issues of either conceptual or geographic boundaries. Nationalism is as much concerned with gaining more territory for the sake of greater security as it is with protecting what the group already possesses. Historical examples help us understand the dynamics of the imperialism and expansionism apart from their pejorative connotations.

From the late 19th century through the time of national socialism, German nationalism grew from a movement dedicated toward a consolidated *Klein Deutschland* to one toward an all-encompassing *Gross Deutschland,* which would contain all "Aryan" peoples. The *Anschluss* whereby Germany annexed Austria in 1938 was a step in that direction. The political act was secondary to the psychological sense of union that underlay it. On one level, the term *Anschluss* might be a metaphor for all deeply felt reunions of racial, ethnic, or national siblings in the family of nationalist sentiment.

Hans Kohn (1960) documented in his work on Pan-Slavism the Slavic nationalists' expanding sense of affiliation. Many of the minority problems in Czecho-Slovakia are attributable to the vicissitudes of ethnonationalist expansion within the borders of post-1918 Czecho-Slovakia. Alas, even the choice of spelling the name reveals the people's loyalties, since Czechs insist on *Czechoslovakia,* aspiring to include Slovak identity in their own, whereas Slovaks seek to establish internal Slovak autonomy while absorbing Ruthene (Rusyn) and non-Ruthene Byzantine-Catholic populations of Slovakia.

Russia has tried to expand Russian identity by incorporating the Ukrainians, who insisted on ethnonational separateness—and tried to absorb Ruthenians into the Ukrainian orbit. Rusyns have long been divided between those seeking merger with Ukrainian, Slovak, or Russian identity and those seeking independence, which, in turn, would mean that many Ukrainians and Slovaks are really Rusyns. Internal nationalist attempts to gain homogeneity by various reforms (e.g., linguistic) also reflect an internal irredentist desire to absorb all who should belong. Lorant Czigany's paper (1974) on the vicissitudes of "Hungarianness" in Hungary illustrates this process (see also Suzan, 1973). The ethnonationalist dynamic universally contains the wish to absorb and be absorbed in greater unity, along with fear of the consequences. The ethnonationalist desires merger in a common identity.

Israeli nationalism, for instance, has a global appeal for most Jews. From Theodor Herzl to David Ben-Gurion, political Zionists have emphasized not only that Israel is a Jewish national homeland, but that Jews throughout the diaspora can achieve their identity only by returning there. The boundaries of the present State of Israel do not correspond to those of the Israeli nationalist identity. Many feel that the borders of Israel given in the Bible, granting historical entitlement, indicate the proper extent of Israel psychogeographically rather than do those determined by current political expedience. Gonen writes:

> *Eretz Yisrael,* or the Land of Israel, is the great symbol which in the past propelled Zionists to create a state and which nowadays impels the more fanatic adherents of the Movement for the Complete Land of Israel to cling to the "Western *Eretz Yisrael*" (the land west of the Jordan). As a matter of fact, the symbol of the complete Land of Israel also holds the promise of possession of the "Eastern *Eretz Yisrael*" (what is now the Kingdom of Jordan), a promise which could be fulfilled should this area be occupied by the Israeli army as a result of another war. (1980, p. 116)

He goes on to say that the land of Israel may for some politicians be an internalized symbol, the functioning equivalent of a self-object that can in some instances trigger the kind of narcissistic reactions that cloud political judgment. Moreover, leaders may exploit unconscious ethnicity for political purposes. In referring to completing Israel by expansion, Gonen uses an uncannily apt term, for it is out of a sense of incompleteness that nationalists feel impelled (by means ranging from the ideological to the militaristic) to expand into those territories of the mind and of geography that will restore their sense of wholeness. This dynamic cuts across the nationalism of both great and small; those with a state; those still in social movement but yet lacking a state; and those that correspond to majority and minority populations. Appeals to the realities nationalists cite as grounds for the inerrancy of their ideology and for the moral right they have to what they seek, ought not distract us from those symbolically masked psychological "actualities" (Erikson, 1968) that nationalists wish to implement in reality. Geopolitical expansionism universally has as its object the search for something lost, the quest for one's missing parts or missing parents "out there," the undoing of painful loss, and the averting of annihilation (for expansion is seen as the opposite of annihilation).

Ethnic identities, even founded on primordial sentiments, are not immutable. One hallmark of group identity is instability. Groups threatened with death renew themselves and in the process redefine themselves. This was the case with the Austro-Hungarian Empire, which until 1918 was a conglomerate of ethnic groups (Austrians, Italians, Hungarians, Transylvanians, Poles, Czechs, Slovaks, Romanians, Serbs, Croatians, and Macedonians). Each group came more and more to use land, legends, music, and dance as potent identity symbols in direct proportion to their feeling of being disadvantaged.

During the 18th century Polish magnates precipitated the partition of Poland between Russia, Prussia, and Austria, but in so doing managed, in the name of freedom, to retain their own vast estates and serfs. After Poland disappeared from the map of Europe in 1795, the Polish people revered their country all the more in their beloved Vistula river, they transformed a folk dance into the Mazurka, and took Chopin deeply into their hearts and souls. It took rumblings for equality, liberty, and fraternity originating in the West to help the people unseat their masters.

Each subsequent disturbing historical event in Poland continues to activate new perceptions based on and colored by the old ones. Such words as *Sejm* (the name of the Polish Parliament), freedom, Russia, and Prussia reactivate old hurts, perceptions, and misperceptions. The very words become perceived as offenses. New events seem to be recurrences of the historic past. Those officers who died in the Katyn Forest in 1944 became the personification of earlier martyrs. The Soviet army became the army of Catherine the Great, just as Hitler's army reactivated the memory of the Prussian role in Poland's dismemberment. Each such event represents a kind of historical transference.

Yugoslavia is a country with fierce antagonisms among its minorities, who not only have disparate ethnic allegiances but different religions and ambitions for separatism. The Croatians, Serbs, Slovenes, Herzegovinians, Montenegrinos, and Macedonians all historically had intense hatred for their neighbors, but under Tito, during the Hitler period, they adapted to the crisis that jarred their previous perceptions of themselves and their counterparts and joined forces. Hitler then became "the other," the target for scapegoating. No people fought with more determination and dedication than the Yugoslavs under Tito, and their adaptive perception lasted as long as Tito lived, although renewed rumblings of discontent and intergroup scapegoating are now appearing.

Intergroup Perspectives

Gregory Bateson (1972) defines information as any difference that makes a difference in the system of which it is a part. Information in ethnic systems is defined as what creates and sustains the differentiation of groups and strengthens group self- and object representation. Cultural information serves the crucial splitting that leads to what Jerome Frank (1967) calls "the image of the enemy" and what Bronfenbrenner (1961) discusses as "the mirror image" between one's own group and that of the adversary. It underlies also what Spicer (1971) refers to as the "oppositional process" between groups. Stein (1975a, 1977, 1978a, 1984a) discusses this ubiquitous process with respect to Jewish/Gentile history; Soviet/American relations (1982); the "melting pot"/pluralistic "mosaic" dichotomy in the ideology of the White Ethnic movement (Stein, 1974a; Stein & Hill, 1973, 1977a, 1977b); and psychologist/psychiatrist professional identities (Stein, Stanhope, & Hill, 1981); the identity of family medicine (Stein, 1981); and a theory of culture and ethnicity (Stein, 1975b, 1980).

We believe that what Lyman Wynne (1965, pp. 298–299) says of the "traded dissociations" between members of pathological families obtains precisely for those governing the interethnic and international family. We find in this a remarkable congruence of individual psychology and group psychology. He holds that "each person sees himself as having a specific limited difficulty which he feels derives from another family member" and thinks that that member is the only person who can alleviate his distress. The latter fails to see how he has contributed to it but is at the same time aware of problems of his own similarly unacknowledged by the first, or another, family member he believes contributes to it. "Thus", notes Wynne, "there is an intricate network of perceptions about others and dissociations about oneself." Each member sees "the totality of a particular quality or feeling in another . . .". Accordingly, the negative view of the other is unmodified by ambivalence, although the presence of the detested quality in the first party in this exchange of dissociation is dissociated out of awareness. "The fixed view that each person has of the other is unconsciously exchanged for a fixed view of himself held by the other."

Wynne notes that he is referring to a system of unconscious processes that permits *each* party to cope with insupportable thoughts and emotions and adds, "The reciprocal . . . trading of dissociations . . . serves to *keep out* of each individual's awareness of himself the dreaded qualities and ideas and also serves to *retain* these qualities within his purview, at a fixed distance from his ego." In this trading of dissociations, each person focuses on whatever the other has but

cannot acknowledge. "Thus, there can be no 'meeting,' no confirmation . . . no shared validation of feelings or experience. Here we
have, of course, an aspect of schizoid and schizophrenic experience."

We emphasize that ethnic groups trade representations of themselves and other groups. That this affects their relationships is often
evidenced in the name calling and language each group uses in
referring to members of another. Even in cultural groups in which
children are taught to abandon individual name calling as uncivil
and immature, it may reappear in adult life as intergroup name
calling when it has group sanction. Reinhold Aman (1981) writes:

> Normally, and world-wide, ethnic groups sharing a common
> border dislike their neighbors and show their dislike or fear
> of them by slurring epithets and proverbs, as Roback's *Diction-*
> *ary of International Slurs* amply proves. The Foreigners' speech
> often is likened to animal sounds or considered no language
> at all. The ancient Greeks, for example, considered the lan-
> guage of their Persian neighbors to the east "barbaric," i.e.,
> "non-Greek, foreign, rough-talking, wild, cruel," just as the
> Poles denounced the language of their German neighbors
> to the west as being no language at all: niemy "mute," whence
> *Niemiec* "German," literally: a mute person. The Malayans liken
> the language of the Tamils to "the rattling of coconuts." When
> American soldiers were first encountered in Germany, in 1945,
> we youngsters made fun of their language by saying that the
> Americans talk as if they had a dumpling in their mouth.
> (pp. 275-276)

Members of a disparaged group are likely to defend themselves
by using the very slurs that their detractors employ against them,
thus identifying with the aggressor and turning passive into active.
The use of "nigger" among blacks, "oilfield trash" among Oklahoma and Colorado roustabouts, and "hunkie" among descendants of Austro-Hungarian immigrants illustrates how common is
this regulation of self-esteem through the adoption of the very
epithets hurled against one's own group.

Ethnic stereotypes and slurs cross continents, oceans, and centuries. Twentieth century Americans and Russians may despise the counterparts they have never seen. To Americans the term *Russian* seems to embody aggressive and dangerous evil. A polarization of "barbarous" Russia and "enlightened" (Western) Europe has dominated European thought for four centuries (Stein, 1976). Nonetheless, local neighbors can also be seen as a chronic threat and focus of identity ambiguity. The "narcissism of minor differences" (Freud, 1930/1961) preserves, even heightens, differences between groups in close proximity. Just as all cognitive categorizing does not serve emotional homeostatic needs, intergroup differences making for intragroup identity and cohesiveness are built around areas of that group's greatest sense of vulnerability and conflict. Difference is felt to be implicit criticism and therefore threatening. Since the objectively small differences so important in the expression of hatred of ethnically different groups are large subjectively, what is at issue is the *perception* of difference rather than absolute difference itself. Minor objective differences grow into subjectively major ones partly to prevent merger with admired but feared out-groups. Large intrapsychic differences needed for defensive purposes appear in such trifling matters as the difference between Russian and Jewish rye bread; in the many names given to the filled pastries of eastern and central Europe—*pirogi, pirohi, piroshki;* and in the ideosyncratic way various Mediterranean groups stuff grape leaves. Each culture boasts of its uniqueness and superiority. The way culture can serve group-narcissism is illustrated by eastern European Jews not only borrowing the potato pancake from the Poles and other Slavs, but changing its Slavic name *oplatek* into the Yiddish *latky* and then claiming that both the dish and its name were indigenous. (These examples are from Stein's work among Slavik-Americans.)

Since the 1960s controversy has raged in American education circles and among minority/ethnic activists (black, Hispanic, Slavic, etc.) over whether differences in cognitive styles or language use between these and mainstream culture were to be construed as "cultural differences" to be respected and nurtured, or whether they were to be construed as "cultural deficits," that is, as signs of something the culture lacked. It seems as if there could be little or no scientific objectivity or detachment on this matter, since to take either position was to offend *someone's* cultural sensibilities. Mainstream American cultural educators and legislators ardently defended the notion of "deficit," arguing variously that English was the bona fide American language, that children of minorities and immigrants needed to acquire American skills that would enable them to succeed in the U.S.A., that *their* parents and grandparents had accommodated to a new cultural milieu and so could the newer groups—all of which had the effect if not intention of asserting and protecting the superiority of mainstream Anglo-American culture.

Educators and spokesmen for various minority cultures argued equally insistently that for a minority group to regard its cultural differences from mainstream culture as deficits would undermine its members' self-esteem and claim to equality as Americans. Protective narcissism became the bane of any effort to compare cultures within the United States and of much remedial or rehabilitative educational policy-making. In defending one's language, one was defending one's "mother tongue," and in turn, one's tie to one's mother and her cultural orbit. Language and culture quickly became embroiled in intergroup competition for status and recognition in the 1960s, 1970s, and 1980s. The object relation-based bipolar split between "good" and "bad" made it insuperably difficult for groups—mainstream and minority alike—to act as if each had something to learn from the other and to value in the other.

A function of ethnic humor is to elevate the status of one's own group by disparaging others. Its ubiquity confirms the notion that narcissistic supplies are limited and that one can raise oneself only by lowering someone else. According to Stanley Brandes (1980):

> One of the most common views about humor and ethnicity is, as Walter Zenner has pointed out, that "it perpetuates negative stereotypes and that it constitutes a form of aggression against the out-group. . . . This view of ethnic humor fits the 'superiority theories' of humor which hold that laughter is directed at those who are considered inferior and is, in itself, a form of triumph and superiority" (1970, p. 93). . . . There is no

doubt that a "limited good" type of mentality (Foster 1967), in which people assume that there exists a finite amount of prestige or esteem in the world, underlies much ethnic joking: if one can deflate one's opponents, albeit only through ridicule and stereotyping, one may correspondingly enhance one's own social status and self-image. (p. 58)

Ethnic humor and other forms of disparagement serve as group homeostats that ensure that the system will remain closed.

In a study of the relationship between tolerance for ambiguity and individuation, Kafka writes that "The developing individual, who must operate in an *open* system, experiences dissonance for which he has not been prepared when his parents operate and communicate as though a *closed* system is the only one in existence" (1971, p. 235). Although he is reexamining double-bind theory, his argument applies to the dynamics of ethnicity since the ideology of ethnonationalist groups and movements tends to insist that an ethnically or nationally closed system is the only emotionally-cognitively tolerable social form. Social distance between groups based on group-specific differences in content serves to overcome any sense of subjective equivalence between groups. Group X and group Y are not subjectively equivalent because one *must* be able to distinguish between them (e.g., Nazis made all Jews, many of whom could not be distinguished from "Aryans" wear arm bands bearing the Star of David; and in the nationalistic American fervor of World War II, Japanese-Americans were interned as enemies in camps because to be Japanese was indisputably to be an enemy).

We rigidly compartmentalize those abstractions (e.g., groups X and Y) between which we are emotionally unprepared to navigate, in order to avoid the uneasiness of ambiguity. With ambiguous intergroup boundaries comes stranger-anxiety, but there is an internal threat also, projected outward as disgust and moral condemnation. For instance, Slovak peasants condemn their Hungarian neighbors and overlords for the overbearingness, arrogance, and cruelty born of a nomadic, equestrian life—but admire their dash from a distance. Conversely, Magyars hold that Slovaks are not human beings, but repulsively sedentary, docile, and passive, thus mirroring the striving that hides beneath their own compensatory ethnic facade. Each clings to the other it needs to hate.

The chronic Jewish dread of the *shiksa* or gentile sirens who, they fear, are certain to seduce loyal Jewish men away from their family traditions is largely projection of a wish. Edwin Friedman (1980), a family therapist, holds that the myth of the *shiksa* has little to do with the way non-Jewish women behave—and virtually everything to do with life within the Jewish family. A man can safely split his ambivalence toward the women of his own group by locating all the feared and taboo qualities outside the group, and all idealized ones within it, as a way of resolving pregenital and oedipal conflicts. He can regard the *shiksa* momentarily as uncanny and hence exotic: what is transiently "me" becomes distinctly "not me." Boundary disputes on cultural no-man's-land occur only at those points at which what is repressed threatens to return to consciousness.

Stein (1980) reexamined Margaret Mead's (1950) rich account of the relationship between the Mountain and Plains Arapesh along the Sepik River of New Guinea, concluding that although the former dissociate hostility from their culture, they exhibit ego- and culture-dystonic aggression by 1) hiring plainsmen to "do their dirty work for them," and 2) projecting all malevolent events in their own society (i.e., illness and death) onto plainsmen. One's cultural adversaries everywhere perform functions essential to the very integrity of the group; indeed, they are psychically inside it though geographically apart.

An example from Stein's work among Slovak-Americans illustrates how ethnicity can be used as a homeostat to ensure changelessness amid rapid social change. In the course of a decade's fieldwork with Slovak-Americans (more generically, Slavic Americans) in western Pennsylvania mill towns, Stein noted an obvious antipathy between Slovaks and blacks. Many pejorative terms were used to describe the latter, who were accused of laziness, untrustworthiness, criminality, sneakiness, shameless breeding, thievery, parasitical behavior, and the like. Stein at first assumed that blacks were a culturally acceptable target upon which Slovaks could externalize unthinkable rebelliousness against their own peasant tradition of repressiveness and inhibition and their dangerous id impulses.

Then he heard several Slovaks refer to blacks and Gypsies in the same way, often interchangeably. "The *Charnyi* (blacks) are American *Czigany* (Gypsies)," said a Slovak in his sixties (November, 1981), who then proceeded to inveigh against American blacks and European Gypsies with equal passion. The inner need to safeguard traditional peasant inhibitions through scorn for a stereotyped out-group was satisfied by the adoption of this new group to embody dissociated group characteristics and to be assigned to the traditional conscious and unconscious matrix (Devereux, 1980, p. 313). Aspects of American culture were "Slovak-ized" or "re-peasantized"; Slovak-Americans came to perceive the host country as recapitulating the old one they had left behind.

Because their contempt both for blacks and Gypsies could be rationalized as being cultural rather than personal, their guilt feelings were minimal: "It's them, not me." The symbolic substitution of black for Gypsy helped bind anxiety associated with unconscionable impulses. Slovak-Americans found in the despised yet envied blacks an acceptable outer representation of inner badness to replace the old and no longer available representation. At the same time a reciprocal stereotype of Slovak-Americans as good, thrifty, industrious, patient, obedient, dependable, responsible, clean, and sexually well controlled was created. To embody only these admirable characteristics, it was necessary to find other people to embody the characteristics they rejected. This example supports the view that psychic structure and social structure are both implemented by projective identification.

An example from recent history illustrates the same process. During the time of national socialism in Germany (1933–45), the name of Felix Mendelssohn became unmentionable, and his music was played only without attribution. His statue at the Gewandhaus in Leipzig was taken down; as a Jew he could not be included within the boundary of what was "Aryan" or German. (Extermination was, of course, the most radical form of ethnic exclusion.)

Reciprocally, none of Wagner's music was performed publicly in Israel after 1948 (although recordings continued to be sold) until Zubin Mehta, conducting the Israel Philharmonic, gave the *Prelude* and *Liebestod* from *Tristan and Isolde*, which prompted a disturbance in the concert hall. Just as Mendelssohn could not be integrated within the affective concept of a Nazi state, likewise Wagner could not be assimilated but became a toxic substance to be expelled or extruded from the post-World War II Jewish state (even though his music had been performed in Palestine through the 1930s). Mendelssohn reminded (represented for) Nazis about what was hateful about Jews; Wagner reminded (represented for) Israelis about what was hateful about Germans. It should be noted, however, that the reciprocity was not symmetrical as Wagner was in fact anti-Semitic.

Erikson (1968, pp. 80–81) claimed that the "exclusiveness of totalism" and the "inclusiveness of wholism" are mutually exclusive. In totalistic identities, whether idiosyncratic or shared, parts of the self not possible to acknowledge as internal (introjects) are externalized. The psychic compromise that accomplishes this lies in the fact that one creates distance from this introject yet preserves a strong symbiotic tie to it. One remains emotionally wedded to it despite conscious divorce.

In his study of the conflict between Turkish and Greek Cypriots, Volkan (1979) observes:

> Cypriot Turks make Cypriot Greeks the target of their externalization of "all bad" self- and object-presentations. Such externalization permits the Turks to keep for their kind all of the "all good" constellations in a rather cohesive way. By way of displacement the Turkish child can distance himself psychologically from the Greeks so completely that he need not mend the split in his perception of external objects around him as being tinged with either Turkish or Greek reference. (1979, p. 63)

The Cypriot Greeks can thus be discounted. Volkan observes that Turkish Cypriots help to repress their incestuous strivings by displacing the incest taboo onto a prohibition of intermarriage with Greek Cypriots.

> When the child brings pregenital problems into the Oedipal phase, "togetherness" with the mother heightens incestuous desires. The energy needed to repress such desires is taxed by the energy demands of a continuation of primitive splitting, and the displacement of the incest taboo on intermarriage provides relief. Thus the social customs of the island support the psychological distancing and primitive splitting that keep the two ethnic groups on the island from merging. And the interplay between established social custom and psychological modes of life is, of course, reciprocal. (1979, p. 64)

One thereby does not feel anguish over oedipal strivings, since it is Cypriot Greeks one would not want to marry, not one's own Cypriot Turkish mother. Preoedipal closeness with the mother can thus be almost indefinitely protracted without oedipal contamination. The reciprocal, social group-role of Cypriot Greek and Cypriot Turk is shored up because the opposing group-representation is needed to sustain the in-group self-representation and cohesiveness. The intergroup role is necessary to maintain intragroup roles. One may consciously discount the other group while having an unconscious need for it in order to discount a part of oneself.

In ethnicity what is outside is an externalized representation of and forum for what is inside. Ethnic (and national) groups are highly significant for one another in ways of which neither is conscious. Stein's work on American ethnicity and European nationalism offers an example of how unconscious factors overdetermine the role of a nation-state on the stage of history. The Slovaks and Poles of east central Europe, as well as their descendants in the United States, are closely related in respect to language, political history, religion, ethos, family organization, and personality (Stein, 1978b; Stein & Hill, 1979). In both Slovakia and Poland the national organization established in feudal times was undermined by the centrifugal force of the nobility and by political and military pressure from outside. The ethos of both exalt strength through suffering, and this has influenced at least to some degree the course of political events in east-central Europe. Martyrdom not only indicates superiority but is expected to bring eventual (and paradoxical) victory through defeat. It is is based on an unvoiced premise of what in another context Devereux calls "masochistic blackmail," the goal of which is to "*extort compassion* . . . by an ostentatious display of helplessness" (1980, p. 244).

One might even suggest that the very fragility and vulnerability of the Polish and Slovak nations as geopolitical entities has been fostered as much from within as from without, by projection of the inner personal fantasies and family dramas of the people onto the stage of political reality. In consequence, the outer world both corresponds to the mythic inner world and contributes to its realization; the cultural "family myth" (Ferreira, 1963) edits and falsifies its own reality—the fact that in the 15th century the militaristic kingdom of Poland extended east to Moscow and south to the Black Sea.

Both nations see themselves in art and story as an oppressed mother, often in the icon of a shackled and violated Virgin Mary. Poles refer to their land as "the crucified Christ of the nations" in reference to both the past (tri-partition) and the present (the Soviet Union). Yet beneath the idealization of the generous, self-sacrificing Slavic mother lurks the mother whose generosity is a way to exact eternal indebtedness (Stein, 1974b, 1978b). This symbolic mother imago will not allow her children outside her orbit of dependency and influence and acts as a persecutory figure one dare not leave lest she abandon one. Her self-abnegation makes the very thought of separation guilty. Her protest "What would you do without me?" is in fact a desperate cry of "What would I do without you?"

The universal early split between mother imagos is often amplified in Slovak and Polish families. In the early family experiences of their children these two mother images are split into a romanticized one that remains conscious and another, unconsciously entertained, that is persecutory and intrusive. The latter, transformed and projected onto national and international perceptions and strategies, may prevent Slovakia or Poland from being internally unified, since the personal and interfamilial ambivalence has not been resolved; self- and object-representations have not been unified in the individual.

Early swaddling, whether or not it creates emotional constriction, is designed to toughen the infant allowed to cry its heart out without gaining attention. Careful supervision is said to keep the baby from breaking in two. He/she is taught that life is meant for suffering and that the most important lesson in life is to bow to circumstances, hoping for the intercession of Mary and Jesus with an implacable God. Yet the very need to exorcise the child's dependency and weakness and to convert it through denial and reaction formation into resilience, endurance, patience, and strength assumes inherent helplessness from which it must but cannot escape, because it must continue to depend on the mother from whom, as from God, "all blessings flow." The symbolic reality of Slovak and Polish nationhood, national history, and national destiny are greatly overdetermined by those family dramas and their influence on psychosexual development. Family role is subsequently acted out in cultural or national role (Beisel, 1980; Kafka, 1978; Ryan, 1980; Stierlin 1976; Stein, 1978b), which in turn confirms family role. Public manifestations of ethnic nationalism have been much studied, but its less obvious and largely concealed aspects have had little attention. It cannot be accurately assessed in terms of the number of known adherents, its violence, or the cogency of its threat to the status quo. Perhaps what is at issue is the nature of the observer's presuppositions.

Few would dispute that the Afro-American movement of the late 1960s and early 1970s was a bona fide ethnonationalist movement, with its repudiation of whiteness and Americanness, recognition of a lost homeland in Africa, affiliation based on cultural notions of race and origin, the use of such designations as black and Afro-American instead of Negro, distinctive dress (e.g., "Afro" hairstyle or the dashiki). It might, however, be harder to hold ethnonationalism accountable for Verdi's operas and the widespread popularity of his music, although he gave voice to Italian nationalist sentiments, often insufficiently disguised to fool the authorities. *Nabucco, Macbeth, Un Ballo in Maschera,* and *Aida* all express in some way the cry "O patria oppressa" that opens Act 4, Scene 1 of *Macbeth.* Verdi's difficulties with the Italian censors in having his operas staged indicates that they grasped the true sentiments behind the disguises. Only in Florence was *Macbeth* allowed to be staged—and that in 1847, a prerevolutionary year. There was more to Verdi's music than song about olden times. The authorities recognized the subject beneath the display—and displacement (Devereux, 1971).

In homes of American Jews after World War II the holiday of Hanukkah, the Festival of Lights, which occurs during December, became a major festival, although officially it is a minor one, more a popular or folk celebration than a liturgical one. Originally it commemorated a successful Jewish uprising against foreigners; the heightening of Hanukkah's significance in mid-20th-century America must be understood in connection with and opposition to the Christian feast of Christmas. Traditionally, only a ritual candle-lighting ceremony with indoors games at home, it is now celebrated with many decorations and much gift giving. Many include even a Christmas tree, renamed "the Hanukkah bush." An illustration of what Devereux and Loeb (1943) call "anatagonistic acculturation," this ethno-religious heightening of Judaism is inseparable from the Christmas with which it is intended to contrast itself, and against which it is designed to fortify resistance. It is a way of being simultaneously like the host culture and different from it. The lure of assimilation is neutralized by the adaptation of aspects of the host culture into the idiom of one's own origins. One can in this way engage in gentile customs as long as they seem to take place in a Jewish fashion. However, it should be emphasized that the expression of Jewishness is revivalistic rather than traditional and is now a new cultural means for shoring up the boundary between gentile and Jewish worlds. It can be seen as a quiescent, accommodative form of nativistic ethnicity (Linton, 1943) intended to pose no threat to the host culture.

Ethnonationalism and its Discontents

Ethnonationalist ideology and sentiment are based on the reparative fantasy of fusion with the newly idealized mother (the group as the "good" mother). Attempts are made to ward off anxieties attendant on regression. The wish at the deepest level may be for resymbiosis with the mother, but group interaction and ideology function much like an adolescent gang, being simultaneously a vehicle for *separation* from the family of origin (a bulwark against the symbiotic pull), and an object for renewed *merger* with a newly idealized "good" object (in contrast with early internalized "bad" objects and conflictual relationships). Ethnonationalism thus has the dual psychic function of loosening early object ties and reestablishing idealized ones through contemporaries. One can thereby have one's cake and eat it, possessing the newly redefined past without being engulfed by it.

Ethnonationalism newly negotiates a "satellite state" (Özbek & Volkan, 1976), wherein one is able to orbit at a safe distance from early objects. One's group of contemporaries serves simultaneously as a bulwark against the past and a reinstatement of the past in acceptable form. As a group compromise formation it satisfies regressive yearnings while forestalling regression to one's actual childhood condition. One thereby metaphorically regains a lost paradise without having to go through the hell of persecution.

The cult of the "good" mother is also that of the "good" father. Through primitive splitting, the "good" father of ethnonationalist fantasy is strong, protective, kind, and forgiving. The "bad" father projected onto the dominant out-group (e.g., WASPs, the USA) is oppressive, or alternately weak and inconsequential, punitive, stern, and castrating. The terrorizing oedipal father who threatens to cut one off from mother is ejected from within the self- and group imago. Just as the all-good mother imago is retained within the group boundary and the all-bad is located within outside adversaries, the all-good father imago is kept, while the all-bad is discovered to be the exclusive property of the world outside the group.

Winnicott's (1965) useful distinction between the protective, nurturant "environment" mother and the exciting, affectionate "sensuous" mother is one we might extend to the father as well. Clearly, in ethnonationalist sentiment, both threatening maternal and paternal fantasies, preoedipal and oedipal, are allocated to the environment outside the ethnonational boundary—or, transitionally, are seen as embodiments of "foreign elements" or "alien contaminants" within the group that must be purged to restore its purity.

It should be emphasized that the ethnic and national solution to the sense of fragmentation is an heroic effort to rescue the idealized traditional nuclear and extended family. One might think of the television series "Father Knows Best" of the 1950s and "The Waltons" of the 1970s and early 1980s as examples of this fantasy in popular culture. Since the "perfect" family is neopatriarchal, Americans look for a strong male head of the American household who "knows best." The choice of Ronald Reagan as president symbolizes this. Many white ethnics vacillate between *spurning* the United States as a land that has abandoned, abused, and oppressed ethnic peoples and *reinventing* it as a pluralistic multiethnic nation—that is, changing the U.S. from being a "bad" father/mother into a good one. With the latter position, according to which one expands the *ethnic* metaphor into a *national* one, the ethnonationalist individual becomes an intensely patriotic American and ascribes feelings of "bad"ness, deprivation, and threat to the Soviet Union, China, Cuba, Iran, and the like. The illusion of complete harmony within the group would seem to require the sowing of discord and conflict with targets of projective identification outside the group. Stated baldly, the price of "peace" is "war."

In viewing ethnonationalism as a process in search of structure rather than as a fixed social entity, we can apply John Hughlings Jackson's (1932) distinction between the dissolution of higher cerebral functions in the formation of the psychoses (the "negative signs") and restitution at more primitive mental functioning (the "positive signs"). The study of ethnonationalism lets us observe and analyze the process of group *dis*organization and *re*organization, which is to say, the loss and regaining of the world. The desperate, panic-stricken quest for "secure boundaries" or "secure borders" is a psychogeographic and psychopolitical representation of the fear of imminent annihilation as the boundaries of the self are felt to collapse. One averts the "internal catastrophe" only by a radical splitting of "good" and "bad" aspects of the self. It is only much later that a more cohesive and stable self- and object-representation congeals.

6

SOME IMPLICATIONS AND RECAPITULATIONS

At the moment of birth man is thrust from intrauterine union into a world of dichotomy, self and other. From this stage of life a prime objective of growth is to distinguish self from other. But simultaneously, dependent needs compel contradictory reunion with mother (the prototypal other) thus inducing ambivalence. Parents then naturally divide and redirect their children's ambivalence, finding good within the family and bad outside. This precedent sets the stage for society to do the same not only with its individuals, but also on the group level.

The faculty of individuals to reunite and fuse with the group appears to be a deeply embedded behavior that assures the survival of the individual, the group, and therefore the species. The faculty is most exercised in times of danger, and then the structure of the family, the community, and their ethnicity all determine the defensive reunification. The Arabs say, "My brother and I against our cousins, we and our cousins against the world." The scale varies but there is ultimately a dichotomy. In ancient times the manner in which Cretan towns abandoned their internecine wars to unite against the common enemy prompted the Greeks to give us the word syncretism. The word may have been archaic and most used by theologians to refer to the amalgamation of different religions, but the political principle endures.

World history for the past two millenia is filled with the lively and deadly flux of nations emerging, growing, prevailing, and succumbing. While the numbers of nations playing the game have grown, there has been a countervailing tendency through alliances to reduce the number of contestants. As the scale of human conflict and all its attributes of destructive power have accelerated in this century, we find ourselves propelled into a world dividing in two. There is still some room for communal and regional strife, but more and more the polarization of the two superpowers imposes itself on us, the species. In our rational moments we flinch at this and its associated nuclear madness, yet we ourselves contribute to it.

Within each of us in some degree lies the need to dichotomize, to externalize unacceptable aspects of ourselves onto the other— the need to have an enemy. It seems that only in fantasy can we envision a scenario in which the world's two blocs might make their peace and unite against the common enemy of another planet. Perhaps the appeal of the star war theme of science fiction and comic books can be understood as a manifestation of the ubiquitous and perpetual need to have an enemy.

The long history and universality of man's need for an enemy, both individually and collectively, compels us to ponder its possible benefits. Perhaps from an evolutionary standpoint it has been a highly adaptive life force. Certainly, some of the mental mechanisms involved (projection, externalization, and denial) relieve anxiety for the individual in daily life. At the group level they may have an analogous anxiety ridding or shielding function even when—and perhaps especially when—they issue in war. So far mankind, as armies, as nations, and as a whole, has been able to afford the cost of the suffering and loss of life. This has been true even as wars grew bigger and more destructive; even in our greatest wars there were many more survivors than fallen. But now, the new and totally different nuclear physics of destruction makes possible a similarly new and totally different human result, namely, the destruction of the species, not just an "acceptable" level of casualties.

Man knows but doesn't fully know this yet, and doesn't know how to accommodate to it. He goes on about his international relations using the same political moves and mental mechanisms he always has. He is confirmed in this habit by the observation that there are plenty of local and regional conflicts that can be and still are played by the old rules and psychological assumptions. There are still some opportunities to externalize badness, to find all evil in the other side, and to destroy it. But it can't be done with nuclear weapons; as we are all coming to realize, this would be suicide. Even in psychological terms it would represent a failure of externalization as the nuclear holocaust would destroy the good internal objects along with the bad external objects. So we may wonder if what has been adaptive for all of man's history may now no longer be so. A change to a new order in physics now demands a change to a new order of psychology.

It is at one level a logical incongruity and at a deeper unconscious level a felt dire necessity that the preservation of abstract ethnicity becomes more important than the preservation of one's life or even the life of the species itself. Here, if we may use a clinical analogy, ethnicity has far more of the quality of a character disorder than a neurotic conflict. For one's ethnicity and its associated magical beliefs are egosyntonic, whereas in neurotic conflict the unacceptable ideas and wishes are ego-dystonic. War is therapeutic in the sense that it consists of a heroic effort to protect the integrity of the character structure. The nuclear madness poses the contradiction that one cannot safeguard the character structure while endangering the species.

Paradoxically, an essential part of conflict resolution with respect to ethnicity is the creation of internal conflict which would interrupt the vicious cycles of externalization and military action based upon this externalization. By transforming ego-syntonicity into ego-dystonicity, ethnicity would become less noxious.

Experience with psychotherapy shows that the first and essential step in dealing with character pathology is the reduction of ego-syntonic character defense and experiencing in its place ego-dystonic conflict. At the social level this need not involve excessive self-doubt, "knocking America," or any form of social betrayal. Societal self-examination and criticism wouldn't have to mean throwing out the baby of loyalty and humanism with the bath water of ethnonationalism. At least in its more extreme expressions, ethnicity would be recognized to be more of a problem than a solution. Optimally, one would be able to say, "I have a problem" or "We have a problem" instead of "You are my problem." By stimulating inner questioning, we stand the chance of conflict resolution or at least the diminution of dangerous externalizing defenses. One would need the external enemy less when one is increasingly able to recognize and come to terms with the enemy within.

There is growing appreciation that the ardent defense of one's ethnonationalism and the nuclear madness have become deeply intertwined. True, the nuclear confrontation under the influence of the impersonal forces of power politics, economics, and rival ideologies has become institutionalized. It is a fixture in the world's life that offers no promise of going away on its own, only of growing. Though it is a human creation, its momentum of growth now seems to be built in and autonomous. But with some countervailing force man recognizes the need to rein in this runaway, this latter-day expression of his age-old disposition to war. Achieving this goal may be aided by returning to and remembering the deeply personal and ethnonational roots of the conflict that underlies the nuclear confrontation.

An important early contribution to this process was made by the Group for the Advancement of Psychiatry in a monograph entitled *Psychiatric Aspects of the Prevention of Nuclear War* (GAP, 1964). Among the many issues dealt with were the problems of dehumanization and mutual distrust. It discussed the need for rehumanization of the problem and considered at length the prospects of international "conflict without violence."

As man seeks to awaken himself to the dangers of his divisive and warlike disposition, all areas of life must participate—individual, social, educational, institutional, and political. We believe everyone can contribute to the eventual success, the more so as we understand ourselves better.

Much of what we have to say about the metapsychology of object relations is familiar to our fellow behavioral scientists. Much of our application of it to an understanding of identity formation in the individual and the group may appear to be hypothetical and strained. In some degree we share this assessment. Paradoxically, to others much of what we have to say may not appear to have broken new ground but seem banal and common knowledge—though dressed up in fancy terms. We would again agree, since some of what we have to say has in essence been said before, both more elegantly and simply, by philosophers and poets such as John Donne, whom we quote. Few will be surprised to hear that man and mankind are one. But we hope we have shed some light on the psychology of the ways in which man and fellowman are one and the ways in which primal fears in clever mutations suspend reason to divide man and men.

This Report places us far closer to the Stoics than to the Utopians. For it is clear that, our most fervent wishes for international peace notwithstanding, all things are not possible for the human animal. Unambivalent love—whether for a person, a family, a work group, a church, or a nation—proves to be a dangerous illusion; hateful feelings, wishes, and ideas that cannot be included in that love must surface somewhere. And where they do so with unrelenting force is in that carefully guarded condensation that Jerome Frank (1982) calls the "image of the enemy." How ironic it is that we do evil in order that we not see and feel ourselves to be evil. A further irony is, that we must come to recognize that what have heretofore been accepted as virtually sacred cultural solutions are themselves contributory to the problem.

The problem of human aggression—whether American or Soviet, Israeli or Palestinian, Turkish or Greek—will not be solved by the defeat of the enemy. But such contrasting lofty philosophical aspirations as internationalism, cosmopolitanism, and universal peace can only be realistically pursued if we can acknowledge that a part of being human has always been the search for an enemy to embody, temporarily or permanently, disavowed aspects of ourselves. These issues must be constantly conscious in the very process of political negotiation, for in that respect, at least, every historic enemy is very much like ourselves.

Writers of tracts such as this—no less than good poets such as Donne—have their prescriptive moment. And once again we may be found trite, echoing the long familiar injunction "know thyself."

This obligation must be met not only at the level of interpersonal relations, but also in the individual discharge of our public responsibilities. Every group—social, work, religious, and so on—to which an individual belongs offers this opportunity for applied insight. The ultimate challenge is to a nation's electorate, whether they be the multitude of a democracy or the few of an oligarchy, to exercise judgment in the selection of leaders who personify the healing spirit rather than partisan polarization. Refining our judgment in this respect comes from the conscious effort to explore the conflicting dispositions to heal and split that lie within each of us, and the ways in which we project them on the world around us.

The adaptive benefits of patriotism, ethnicity, nationalism, and similar expressions of group belonging are indisputable. To challenge them is like challenging motherhood. Indeed, given our views on the continuity and unity of man, motherhood and patriotism are of the same piece. The nobility of the ultimate expressions of love and self-sacrifice in patriotism as in motherhood make challenge sacrilegious. But realistically we know motherhood miscarries, and sins are committed in its name. Samuel Johnson only reminded us of what we know when he referred to patriotism as the last refuge of a scoundrel. Too often it is similarly misused as the first plank in the politician's platform. A leader's need to appeal to the essential unity between himself and his group often identifies him as follower more than leader, currying favor rather than enlightening. No State of the Union message is made without innumerable "My fellow Americans." It is encouraging then to hear an American president, at least in one State of the Union message, reach out and address the Russians—other citizens of the planet.

In a democracy the dialectic of the dance of the leader and the people is one of short steps; neither partner can get much ahead of the other. Unfortunately, in the present state of the world the people appear to be offering cues in favor of peace and nuclear disarmament, which their leaders seem unable to act upon. The balance between the needs of peace and those of self-defense is kept close by adherence to traditional views of what constitutes national self-defense. Self-defense has ever been common sense.

Now, however, the nuclear danger suggests that there may be circumstances in which national self-defense does not make sense. Or at least a new perspective that takes into account the species as a whole is required.

Fortunately our new world is not entirely lacking in leaders capable of a transcendent new world vision. Nor do we lack leaders of sufficient personal ego capacity and maturity to forego the "natural" inclination to respond to group-humiliations and defeats with retaliatory shame-reversing aggression. In recent history, for instance, Soviet Premier Nikita Khrushchev (in response to President Kennedy's blockade of Cuba in 1962) seemed to exemplify a leader who was able to absorb shame and respond maturely. President Kennedy rejected Soviet leader Khruschev's proposal to exchange Soviet missiles in Cuba for American ones in Turkey. Accused of cowardice by his military advisors, Khrushchev was able to forego the more automatic response of retaliatory shaming against the U.S. Khrushchev later wrote of his advisors:

> They looked at me as though I was out of my mind or, what was worse, a traitor . . . The biggest tragedy, as they saw it, was that the Chinese or Albanians would accuse us of weakness. I said to myself: To hell with these maniacs . . . What good would it have done me in the last hour of my life to know that though our great nation and the United States were in complete ruin, the national honor of the Soviet Union was intact? (quoted in Cousins, 1977, p. 4)

Inextricably tied to leadership, there is the issue of avoiding inter*group* humiliation in the wake of military and political defeat. Whatever one might observe of German national character continuities over the centuries (Dundes, 1984), it is insufficient to ascribe the entire responsibility for the horrors of 1933–1945 to Germany alone. A number of professional historians have advanced the retrospective argument that Allied vindictiveness, expressed in punitive "reparative" measures against Germany, created such economic hardship that Germany was provoked to belligerent redress. Perhaps Versailles came too soon after the dreadful suffering of the Allies to expect any measure of understanding, never mind compassion, for German society and history. But we may speculate that some understanding and more lenient peace terms might have mitigated the strident vengeance of the German people in their grotesque attempts to restore group self-esteem. This particular lesson of history was not lost on the Allies in writing peace terms after World War II; and the close alliance of Germany and Japan with the West no doubt supports this contention. It is, however, regrettable that the principle of the lesson has been lost in relation to the Soviet Union. Lack of appreciation for the Soviet contribution in winning World War II and failure to acknowledge their suffering in that conflict injures their self-esteem and sharpens their hostility to the West.

We know the world is a dangerous place, so it is natural and proper that every leader take seriously the defense of his community. We would not ask that leaders be out of step with their people, but we can ask that they take the steps people cannot take individually. Now nuclear weapons compel us—as we have here attempted—to redefine the community. Leadership of the superpowers is in the hands of older men whose vision of the world is "prenuclear." The problem is not that they can't see the danger; they see it quite clearly and rationally. The problem lies in the inability of the clear and rational realization to alter the whole set of mental representations that constitute the world view of these leaders. These mental representations are composed of so much material that is forgotten or half-forgotten, loaded with affect and instinct, tinged with factual inaccuracy, and so dearly held that new information and reason make only slow progress. The leader whose adolescent concept of warfare was shaped by Spitfires and B29s may know at one level that nuclear war would be different, but much of his mental life is under the sway of earlier concepts, images, and emotions.

Such mental sets are not readily changed, but some modification can be achieved by putting oneself in the other person's shoes. Freeman Dyson (1984) has argued in favor of a conscious effort to identify ourselves with the Soviet people.

> It is important for Americans to go through the mental exercise of looking at nuclear weapons as if they had been Hitler's weapons rather than ours, because this exercise enables us to come closer to seeing nuclear weapons as they are seen by Soviet citizens. To understand Russian strategy and diplomacy, it is necessary for us to distance ourselves from our own myths and to enter into theirs. An understanding of Soviet views is the essential first step toward any lasting amelioration of the danger in which the world now stands.

This exercise is somewhat analogous to the anticipatory fantasy that many people have found helpful in preparing to deal with expected problems of living.

If we take the last few millennia as a guide, we would be foolhardy to expect major changes in human object relations during the next few thousand years. Freud (1932) in his correspondence with Einstein found some hope—though he feared it was Utopian—in the education of "an elite of independent thinkers." Such an elite would, we may hope, accomplish basic changes in their own views and attitudes toward intergroup and international relations. Changes away from externalization, projections, and similar mental mechanisms might then parallel at the societal level those that can occur in individual psychotherapy.

A sort of trickle-down effect in society may be expected from psychoanalytic psychology and its cognate psychodynamic therapies. Acting in concert with a psychodynamically informed educational system, they could certainly contribute to a lessening of emotional vulnerability in succeeding generations, and would thus constitute something of a preventive measure to decrease the risk of aggression in defense of one's ethnicity. This might, for example, work in the following manner: For parents and other early caregivers, the infant and child is itself an "object" of care-givers' need to exteriorize idealized and unacceptable parts of their selves. Since the child is used as a container defensively, so to speak, to help the care-givers shore up their own selves and higher defenses, to the degree to which these adults can be helped to work through their early object relations vicissitudes and conflicts, they will lessen their inner burden upon the next generation and thereby make the child less vulnerable to using primitive defenses when group-stress occurs.

Maturational change of the superego entails a structural change that makes possible a recognition of the other as an animate center of experience and action. This implies more than mere ability to identify with the other; it implies the ability to shift perspective on what comprises humanity. Here we are referring to a view of the human species as one organism, a view that transcends the limited horizon of our group as the true species and the other gang as pseudospecies.

The world is a dangerous place and lonely man is constantly driven to seek safety in his community through the regressive merging that issues in ethnicity, nationalism, and various "Pan-isms." This current trend represents a remarkable contrast to the unifying movements that marked the earlier years of this century, when internationalism was the ideal and we were all to learn to speak Esperanto. Once the ideal was to do away with ethnicity, now it is to find the ideal ethnicity.

Attached to this kind of illusory hope there is now a still more irrational hope of security in our nuclear arms and a magical defense against theirs. We speak of nuclear madness and it is not an empty epithet or metaphor. Actual nuclear conflict could be the ultimate self-destructive expression of man's psychotic side.

The moment of death is difficult for the ego to face, even for normal man facing normal death. But as anxious and dysphoric as may be the feelings that attend this dissolution of the ego, there is a much worse torment. It is the absolute loneliness and nothing-ness associated with psychosis, psychotic panic, and psychotic world destruction fantasies and delusions. These psychological experi-ences sometimes erupt in actions such as mass murders, massacres, and terrorism. They often involve the perpetrator's self-destruction, thus achieving a paradoxical escape from the psychotic agony. It is conceivable that in some circumstances nuclear weapons might find a place in these actions. Indeed, we must ponder the possibility that the very power of nuclear weapons might tempt, reinforce, and elicit such impulses and behavior among desperate leaders. Though Adolph Hitler might not be considered clinically psychotic, we may wonder if world destruction impulses may have moved him to order the burning of Paris as his forces retreated and then a scorched earth policy even in his own Germany, which would have destroyed the German people had he not been disobeyed. It is both frightening and salutory to contemplate what might have happened if Hitler possessed nuclear weapons in our current abundance.

So, as the world is a dangerous place, man lives in his village. He finds comfort and security there and in peaceful times all may admire and enjoy the cultural diversity of the world's many villages. A hopeful evolution of the species' course is that we may come to terms psychologically with our inhabiting a global village, and that our lapses into ethnonational madness may prove to be only temporary regressive phenomena along the path of our progress. To ask the world's villages to give up their diversity and speak only Esperanto would be too much and too dull. But we may reasonably ask the villagers to learn the psychological Esperanto of man's unities and divisions.

Recapitulation

The experience of being connected with an ethnic or national group often enhances self-esteem and provides a source of strength for the individual and the group. It becomes problematical and sometimes dangerous when it serves as a focal point of vulnerabilities and even pathology—whether those of the individual or the group. Our concern over the all too frequent destructive effects of ethnonationalism prompted this psychological study, which we hope will contribute modestly to understanding this very human issue.

Ethnonationalistic attitudes have their origins in biology and the individual's infantile experiences of self-other differentiation. Within a few years self-other differentiation at the group level is established in the context of families, schools, racial differences, and so on. The resulting differences—however accurately or inaccurately perceived—are crystalized in adolescence by the ongoing formation of identity and character that marks that phase of life. Particular cultural circumstances provide common denominators of characteristics that are shared by numerous individuals. In this way basic human feelings and needs are experienced in group contexts, therefore providing reservoirs of attitudes that are available to shape group behavior under the influence of leaders.

Though wary of being prescriptive, we believe this Report— centered around these salient points—can help educators, public officials, and other leaders to detoxify the noxious aspects of ethnonationalism without losing its integrative and cultural benefits.

1. Under stressful circumstances individuals and peoples may react constructively, but they may also regress to early-life modes of reaction including *dichotomizing and splitting* the social world into "good" or pleasurable feelings, thoughts, and people (that is, "us" and our friends) and "bad" or unpleasurable feelings, thoughts, and people (that is, "them," the enemies). Especially under stress, people overvalue and overemphasize sameness within their group and differences between themselves and their adversaries.

2. The concept of the *"Enemy"* is not simple—and not an entirely separate entity. The American concept of "Russianness," for example, does not consist solely of what Russians are, but contains some of our own unwanted parts which have been externalized and projected onto Russians in psychological patterns, which we explore. (As these phenomena are universal, the Russians of course do the same with us.) Part of this psychology is that the dissociated parts of "us" that have been implanted in "them" must not be completely discarded but must be retained at a safe distance. So negotiating with "them" entails, in addition to the conscious agenda, negotiating with parts of "us." This often unconscious symbiosis between adversaries is a powerful factor in human negotiations.

3. *Unconscious contaminants* complicate and cloud the assessment of objective circumstances in intergroup relations. Ethnonationalism is often a sanctioning cloak under which the boundaries

between the abstract and the concrete may be confounded. Culture, ritual, psychogeography, and so on may be so distorted, that it is difficult to arrive at the "reality" of one's own boundaries and vulnerability. The corollary is of course a misperception of the enemy threat, vulnerability, and so forth.

4. Some features of ethnonationalism may be considered irrational or even "crazy." In this Report we identify certain processes and structures of the mind that make it possible for these features to coexist with reason and sanity.

People inhabit different assumptive or representational worlds. They consider their own world to be right and sane, others' intrinsically wrong, "crazy," and dangerous. A rational approach to these *irrational or pseudoirrational worldviews* must avoid scornful political and ideological postures that challenge the human worth of the adversary, along with the colorations of his assumptive world. Patience, tact, and careful timing are the sine qua non of any effort to change human conviction—especially nonrational convictions.

5. "Us" and "them" polarization tends to be self-perpetuating and impedes change, within the self and within the others we wish to change. It interferes with finding a solution to the historical hurts, grievances, and defeats that require acknowledgment, negotiation, *mourning*, and working through. The alternative is continuing hostility, rounds of retaliations, and the transmission of historical enmity to future generations. This emerges as an area of particular responsibility for leaders.

6. *Leaders* are necessary personifications of group history, present political process, and aspirations for the future. Being expressions of the group, they are far less autonomous than widely shared nonpsychological viewpoints would suggest. Still, in the dialectic of leaders and groups, there is an important place for individuality and initiative. The influence of leaders is as double edged as the sword of ethnonationalism itself. They have the opportunity to help their people mourn, heal, and overcome group hurt or to perpetuate hurt and to destroy— albeit in the name of preserving the purity and goodness of their groups.

BIBLIOGRAPHY

Aman, R. (1981). "They are a hairy, cruel, savage nation": Ethnic slurs anno 1774. *Maledicta, 5,* 273-283.

Barnes, F.F. (1980). Travel and fatigue as causes of partial dissociative reactions. *Comprehensive Psychiatry, 21*(1), 55-61.

Barth, F. (Ed.). (1969). *Ethnic groups and boundaries.* Boston: Little, Brown & Co.

Bateson, G. (1972). *Steps to an ecology of mind.* San Francisco: Chandler.

Beisel, D.R. (1980). *Chamberlain and the Munich crisis.* Paper presented at panel on France and Britain in the Development of the Second World War. Third Annual International Psychohistorical Association Convention, New York City, June 12.

Bion, W.R. (1961). *Experiences in groups.* New York: Basic Books.

Blos, P. (1979). Character formation in adolescence. In *The adolescent passage* (pp. 171-191). New York: International Universities Press.

Brandes, S. (1980). *Metaphors of masculinity: Sex and status in Andalusian folklore.* Philadelphia: University of Pennsylvania Press.

Brazelton, T.B., Koslowski, B., & Main, M. (1974). The origins of reciprocity: The early mother-infant interaction (pp. 39-66). In M. Louis & L.A. Rosenblum (Eds.), *The effect of the infant on its caregiver.* New York: Wiley-Interscience.

Bronfenbrenner, U. (1961). The mirror image in Soviet-American relations: A social psychologist's report. *Journal of Social Issues, 17,* 45-56.

Butler, R.N. (1975). *Why survive? Being old in America.* New York: Harper & Row.

Clark, K.B., & Clark, M.P. (1947). Racial identification and preference in Negro children (pp. 169-178). In T.M. Newcomb & E.L. Hartley (Eds.), *Readings in Social Psychology.* New York: Holt.

Cohen, R. (1978). Ethnicity problems and focus in anthropology. *Annual Review Anthropology, 7,* 374-403.

Cota-Robles de Suarez, C. (1973). Sexual stereotypes: Psychological and cultural survival. *Regeneration, 29,* 341-347.

Cousins, N. (1977). The Cuban missile crisis: An anniversary. *Saturday Review,* October 17, p. 4.

Czigany, L.G. (1974). Hungarianness: The origin of a pseudo-linguistic concept. *The Slavonic and East European Review, 52*(128), 325-336.

Deutsch, H. (1944). *The psychology of women: A psychoanalytic interpretation* (Vol. 1 [two volumes]). New York: Grune & Stratton.

Devereux, G. (1955). Charismatic leadership and crisis. In G. Roheim (Ed.), *Psychoanalysis and the social sciences* (Vol. 4, pp. 145-157). New York: International Universities Press.

Devereux, G. (1971). Art and mythology: A general theory. In Carol F. Jopling (Ed.), *Art and aesthetics in primitive societies* (pp. 193-224). New York: E.P. Dutton & Co.

Devereux, G. (1980). *Basic problems of ethno-psychiatry* (B.M. Gulati & G. Devereux Trans.). Chicago: The University of Chicago Press.

Devereux, G., & Loeb, E.M. (1943). Antagonistic acculturation. *American Sociological Review, 8,* 133-148.

DeVos, G. (1975). Ethnic pluralism: Conflict and accommodation. In G. DeVos & L. Komanucci-Ross (Eds.), *Ethnic identity: Cultural continuities and change* (pp. 5-41). Palo Alto: Mayfield.

Dorn, R.M. (1969). Psychoanalysis and psychoanalytic education: What kind of journey? In J.A. Lindon (Ed.), *The psychoanalytic forum* (Vol. 3, pp. 237-274). New York: Science House.

Dundes, A. (1984). *Life is like a chicken coop ladder: A portrait of German culture through folklore.* New York: Columbia University Press.

Dyson, F. (1984). Cutting nuclear myths down to size (Review of *Understanding Weapons in a Nuclear Age* and *The Abolition*). *Science,* June 1984, p. 88.

Emde, R.N., & Harmon, R.J. (1972). Endogenous and exogenous smiling systems in early infancy. *Journal of the American Academy of Child Psychiatry, 11,* 177-200.

Erikson, E.H. (1956). The problem of ego identity. *Journal of the American Psychoanalytic Association, 4,* 56-121.

Erikson, E.H. (1966). Ontogeny of ritualization. In R.M. Lowenstein, A. Solnit, & M. Schur (Eds.), *Psychoanalysis: A general psychology* (pp. 601-621). New York: International Universities Press.

Erikson, E.H. (1968). *Identity: Youth and crisis.* New York: Norton.

Fast, I. (1979). Developments in gender identity: Gender differentiation in girls. *International Journal of Psycho-Analysis, 60,* 443.

Fenichel, O. (1945). *The psychoanalytic theory of neurosis.* New York: Norton.

Ferreira, A.J. (1963). Family myth and homeostasis. *Archives of General Psychiatry, 9,* 55-61.

Foster, G.M. (1967). Peasant society and the image of limited good. In J.M. Potter, M.N. Diaz, & G.M. Foster (Eds.), *Peasant society: A reader* (pp. 300-323). Boston: Little, Brown & Co.

Frank, J. (1967). *Sanity and survival: Psychological aspects of war and peace.* New York: Vantage Books.

Frank, J.D. (1982). Prenuclear-age leaders and the nuclear arms race. *American Journal of Orthopsychiatry, 52*(4):630-637.

Freud, A. (1958). Adolescence. *The psychoanalytic study of the child* (Vol. 13, pp. 255-278). New York: International Universities Press.

Freud, S. (1961). Civilization and its discontents. In J. Strachey (Ed. and Trans.), *The standard edition of the complete psychological works of Sigmund Freud* (Vol. 21, pp. 64-134). London: Hogarth Press. (Original work published 1930)

Freud, S. (1964). Why war? In J. Strachey (Ed. and Trans.), *The standard edition of the complete psychological works of Sigmund Freud* (Vol. 22, pp. 197–215). London: Hogarth Press. (Original work published 1933)

Freud, S. (1964). Splitting of the ego in the process of defence. In J. Strachey (Ed. and Trans.), *The standard edition of the complete psychological works of Sigmund Freud* (Vol. 23, p. 271). London: Hogarth Press. (Original work published 1940)

Friedman, Edwin H. (1980) The myth of the Shiksa. *The Family, 8*(1), 13–22.

Galanter, M. (1981). Cohesiveness in the "large—group": A sociological perspective. In Henry Kellerman (Ed.), *Group cohesion.* New York: Grune & Stratton.

GAP. Committee on Social Issues. (1964). *Psychiatric aspects of the prevention of nuclear war* (Vol. V, Publication No. 57). New York: Mental Health Materials Center, Inc.

GAP. Committee on International Relations. (1978). *Self-involvement in the Middle East conflict* (Vol. X, Publication No. 103). New York: Mental Health Materials Center, Inc.

Geertz, C. (1973). *The interpretation of cultures.* New York: Basic Books.

Geleerd, E.R. (1961). Some aspects of ego vicissitudes in adolescence. *Journal of the American Psychoanalytic Association, 9,* 394–405.

Genet, J. (1960). *The blacks: A clown show.* New York: Grove Press.

Gittler, J.B. (1977). Toward defining an ethnic minority. *International Journal of Group Tensions, 7,* 4–19.

Gonen, J.Y. (1975). *A psychohistory of Zionism.* New York: Mason Charter.

Gonen, J.Y. (1980). Review of *Self-involvement in the Middle East conflict* (Formulated by the Committee on International Relations, Group for the Advancement of Psychiatry, 1978). *Journal of Psychohistory, 8*(1), 111–116.

Goodman, M.E. (1964). *Race awareness in young children.* New York: Collier Books.

Goodman, M.E. (1967). *The individual and culture.* Homewood, IL: The Dorsey Press.

Greeley, A.M. (1974). Political participation among ethnic groups in the United States: A preliminary reconnaissance. *American Journal of Sociology, 80,* 170–204.

Greeley, A.M., & McCready, W.C. (1975). The transmission of cultural heritages in the case of Irish and Italians. In N. Glaser & D.P. Moynihan (Eds.), *Ethnicity: Theory and experience.* Cambridge: Harvard University Press.

Greenacre, P. (1971). The influence of infantile trauma on genetic patterns. In *Emotional growth* (Vol. 1, pp. 260–299). New York: International Universities Press.

Hamilton, J.W. (1966). Some dynamics of anti-Negro prejudice. *The Psychoanalytic Review, 53,* 5–15.

Hamilton, J.W. (1981). Review of C.F. Keyes (Ed.), *Ethnic adaptation and identity: The Karen on the Thai frontier with Burma. American Anthropologist, 83,* 952–955.

Hartley, E.L., Rosenbaum, M., & Schwartz, S. (1948). Children's use of ethnic frames of reference: An exploratory study of children's conceptualizations of multiple ethnic group membership. *The Journal of Psychology, 26,* 367–386.

Isaacs, H. (1975). *Idols of the tribe: Group identity and political change.* New York: Harper & Row.

Jackson, J.H. (1932). The factors of insanity. In *Selected Writings,* (Vol. 1, pp. 411–421). London: Hodder and Stoughton.

Jacobson, E. (1964). *The self and the object world.* New York: International Universities Press.

Jaffe, D.S. (1968). The mechanism of projection. Its dual role in object relations. *International Journal of Psycho-Analysis, 49*, 662-677.

Kafka, J.S. (1971). Ambiguity for individuation: A critique and reformulation of double-bind theory. *Archives of General Psychiatry, 25*, 232-239.

Kafka, J.S. (1978). Review of Helm Stierlin (Author), *Adolf Hitler: A family perspective. Psychiatry, 41*, 221-225.

Kafka, J.S. (1983). Challenge and confirmation in ritual action. *Psychiatry, 46*, 31-39.

Kafka, J.S., & McDonald, J.W. (1965). The latent family in the intensive treatment of the hospitalized schizophrenic patient. In J. Masserman (Ed.), *Current psychiatric therapies* (Vol. 5, pp. 172-177). New York: Grune & Stratton.

Kandel, E.R. (1983). From metapsychology to molecular biology, explorations into the nature of anxiety. *The American Journal of Psychiatry, 140* (12), 1277-1293.

Kernberg, O.F. (1966). Structural derivatives of object relationship. *International Journal of Psycho-Analysis, 47*, 236-253.

Kernberg, O.F. (1976a). Foreword. In V.D. Volkan (Author), *Primitive internalized object relations*. New York: International Universities Press.

Kernberg, O.F. (1976b). *Object relations theory and clinical psychoanalysis*. New York: Jason Aronson.

Klein, M. (1955). On identification. In E. Jaques & B. Joseph (Eds.), *Our adult world and other essays* (pp. 55-98). New York: Basic Books.

Klüver, H. (1936). The study of personality and the method of equivalent and non-equivalent stimuli. *Character and Personality, 5*, 91-112.

Kohn, H. (1960). *Panslavism: Its history and ideology.* New York: Vintage Books.

Kohut, H. (1971). *The analysis of the self: A systematic approach to the psychoanalytic treatment of narcissistic personality disorders.* New York: International Universities Press.

Kohut, H. (1977). *Restoration of the self.* New York: International Universities Press.

Krystal, H. (1974). The genetic development of affects and affect regression. *The Annual of Psychoanalysis, 2*, 98-126.

Krystal, H. (1975). Affect tolerance. *The Annual of Psychoanalysis, 3*, 179-218.

Krystal, H., & Raskin, H.A. (1970) *Drug dependence. Aspects of ego functions.* Detroit: Wayne State University Press.

Kubie, L.S. (1965). The outgoing of racial prejudice. *Journal of Nervous and Mental Diseases, 141*, 265-273.

La Barre, W. (1968). *The human animal.* Chicago: University of Chicago Press.

La Barre, W. (1972). *The ghost dance: The origins of religion.* New York: Dell.

Laplanche, J., & Pontalis, J.B. (1973). *The language of psychoanalysis.* New York: Norton.

Leach, E.R. (1964). *Political systems of highland Burma.* Boston: Beacon Press.

LeVine, R., & Campbell, D. (1972). *Ethnocentrism: Theories of conflict, ethnic atttitudes and group behavior.* New York: John Wiley & Sons.

Levi-Strauss, C. (1963), *Structural anthropology* (Vol. 1). New York: Basic Books

Levi-Strauss, C. (1967). *Structural anthropology* (Vol. 2). New York: Basic Books.

Linton, R. (1943). Nativistic movements. *American Anthropologist, 45*, 230-240.

McDonald, M. (1970). *Not by the color of their skin.* New York: International Universities Press.

Mack, J.E. (1983). Nationalism and the self. *The Psychohistory Review,* *11*(2-3), 47-69.
Mahler, M.S. (1968). *On human symbiosis and the vicissitudes of individuation.* New York: International Universities Press.
Marmor, J. (1966). Nationalism, internationalism, and emotional maturity. *The International Journal of Social Psychiatry, XII*(3), 217-220.
Mead, M. (1950). *Sex and temperament in three primitive societies.* New York: Mentor.
Mejuia, D. (1983). The development of Mexican-American children. In G.J. Powell, J. Yamamoto, A. Romero, & A. Morales (Eds.), *The psychosocial development of minority group children* (pp. 77-114). New York: Brunner/Mazel.
Niederland, W.C. (1956). River symbolism, Part 1. *Psychoanalytic Quarterly, 25,* *469-504.*
Niederland, W.C. (1957). River symbolism, Part 2. *Psychoanalytic Quarterly, 26,* 50-75.
Niederland, W.C. (1971). The naming of America. In M. Kanzer (Ed.), *The unconscious today: Essays in honor of Max Schur.* New York: International Universities Press.
Norton, D. G. (1983), Black family life patterns, the development of self and cognitive development of black children. In G.J. Powell, J. Yamamoto, A. Romero, & A. Morales (Eds.), *The psychosocial development of minority group children* (pp. 181-193). New York: Brunner/Mazel.
Novick, J., & Kelly, K. (1970). Projection and externalization. *The psychoanalytic study of the child* (Vol. 25, pp. 69-95). New York: International Universities Press.
Oxford English Dictionary (Compact Ed.) (1971). New York: Oxford University Press.
Özbek, A., & Volkan, V.D. (1976). Psychiatric problems within the satellite extended families of Turkey. *American Journal of Psychotherapy, 30*(4), 576-582.
Pao, P.N. (1965). The role of hatred in the ego. *Psychoanalytic Quarterly, 34,* 257-264.
Parsons, T., Shils, E., Naegele, K.D., & Pitts, J.R. (1961). *Theories of society* (Vol. 1). Glencoe, IL: The Free Press.
Peterson, W. (1980). Concepts of ethnicity. In *Harvard encyclopedia of American ethnic groups* (pp. 234-242). Cambridge: Harvard University Press.
Pinderhughes, C.A. (1979). Differential bonding: Toward a psychophysiological theory of stereotyping. *The American Journal of Psychiatry, 136*(1):33-37.
Pinderhughes, C.A. (1982). Paired differential bonding in biological, psychological, and social systems. *American Journal of Social Psychiatry, 2*(3), 5-14. New York: Brunner/Mazel.
Powell, G.J., Yamamoto, J., Romero, A., & Morales, A. (Eds.). (1983). *The psychosocial development of minority group children.* New York: Brunner/Mazel.
Proshansky, H.M. (1966). The development of intergroup attitudes. In L.W. Hoffman, & M.L. Hoffman (Eds.), *Review of child development* (Vol. 2, pp. 311-371). New York: Russell Sage Foundation.
Radke, M.J., Trager, H.G., & Davis, H. (1949). Social perceptions and attitudes of children. *Genetic Psychology Monographs, 40,* 327-447.
Reminick, R.A. (1983). *Theory of ethnicity: An anthropologist's perspective.* Washington: University Press of America.
Rice, A.K. (1969). Individual, group, and intergroup processes. *Human Relations, 22,* 565-584.
Rioch, M.J. (1970). The Work of Wilfred Bion and Groups. *Psychiatry* 33:56-66.

Romero, A. (1983). The Mexican-American child: A sociological approach to research. In G.J. Powell, J. Yamamoto, A. Romero, & A. Morales (Eds.), *The psychosocial development of minority group children* (pp. 538-572). New York: Brunner/Mazel.

Royce, A.P. (1982). *Ethnic identity: Strategies of diversity.* Bloomington: Indiana University Press.

Ryan, S. (1980). Petain and Vichy: Abandonment, guilt, "love of harlot," and repetition compulsion. *The Journal of Psychohistory, 8*(2), 149-158.

Sandler, J., & Sandler, A.M. (1978). On the development of object relationships and affects. *International Journal of Psycho-Analysis, 59,* 285-296.

Santos, R.A. (1983). The social and emotional development of Filipino-American children. In G.J. Powell, J. Yamamoto, A. Romero, & A. Morales (Eds.), *The psychosocial development of minority group children* (pp. 131-146). New York: Brunner/Mazel.

Schmale, A.H., Jr. (1964). A genetic view of affects. *The psychoanalytic study of the child, 19,* 287-310.

Searles, H.F. (1965). *Collected papers on schizophrenia and related subjects* (pp. 17-38). New York: International Universities Press.

Shafer, B.C. (1976). *Nationalism: Its nature and interpreters.* Washington, D.C.: American Historical Association.

Shafer, B.C. (1982). *Nationalism and internationalism: Belonging in human experience.* Malabar, FL: Robert E. Drieger Publishing Co.

Shibutani, T., & Kwan, K.K. (1965). *Ethnic stratification: A comparative approach.* New York: Macmillan.

Shils, E. (1957). Primordial, personal, sacred, and civil ties. *British Journal of Sociology, 8,* 130-145.

Spitz, R.A. (1965). *The first year of life.* New York: International Universities Press.

Spicer, E.H. (1971). Persistent cultural systems. *Science, 174,* 795-800.

Stein, H.F. (1974a). Confirmation of the white ethnic stereotype. *School Review, 82*(3), 437-454.

Stein, H.F. (1974b). Envy and the evil eye among Slovak-Americans: An exploration into the psychological ontogeny of belief and ritual. *Ethos, 2*(1), 13-46.

Stein, H.F. (1975a). American Judaism, Israel, and the new ethnicity. *Cross Currents* 25 (1):51-66.

Stein, H.F. (1975b). Ethnicity, identity, and ideology. *School Review, 83,* 273-300.

Stein, H.F. (1976). Russian nationalism and the divided soul of the Westernizers and Slavophiles. *Ethos, 4*(4), 403-438.

Stein, H.F. (1977). The binding of the son: Psychoanalytic reflections on the symbiosis of anti-Semitism and anti-Gentilism. *Psychoanalytic Quarterly, 46,* 650-683.

Stein, H.F. (1978a). Judaism and the group-fantasy of martyrdom: The psychodynamic paradox of survival through persecution. *The Journal of Psychohistory, 6*(2), 151-210.

Stein, H.F. (1978b). The Slovak-American "swaddling ethos": Homeostat for family dynamics and cultural continuity. *Family Process, 17,* 31-45.

Stein, H.F. (1979). The white ethnic movement, Pan-ism, and the restoration of early symbiosis: The psychohistory of a group-fantasy. *The Journal of Psychohistory, 6*(3), 319-359.

Stein, H.F. (1980). Culture and ethnicity as group-fantasies: A psychohistoric paradigm of group identity. *The Journal of Psychohistory, 8*(1), 21-51.

Stein, H.F. (1981). Family medicine as a meta-specialty and the dangers of over-definition. *Family Medicine, 13*(3), 3-7.

Stein, H.F. (1982). Adversary symbiosis and complementary group dissociation: An analysis of the U.S./U.S.S.R. conflict. *International Journal of Intercultural Relations, 6,* 55-83.

Stein, H.F. (1984a). The Holocaust, the uncanny, and the Jewish sense of history. *Political Psychology, 5*(1), 5-35.

Stein, H.F. (1984b). The scope of psycho-geography: The psychoanalytic study of spatial representation. *The Journal of Psychoanalytic Anthropology, 7*(1), 23-73.

Stein, H.F. (1985). Ethnicity, nationalism and internationalism: Review essay. *Journal of Psychoanalytic Anthropology, 8*(1), 81-87.

Stein, H.F., & Hill, R.F. (1973). The new ethnicity and the white ethnic in the United States: An exploration in the psycho-cultural genesis of ethnic irredentism. *The Canadian Review of Studies in Nationalism, 1*(1), 81-105.

Stein, H.F., & Hill, R.F. (1977a). *The imperative: Examining the new white ethnic movement.* University Park, PA: The Pennsylvania State University Press.

Stein, H.F., & Hill, R.F. (1977b). The limits of ethnicity. *The American Scholar. 46*(2), 181-189.

Stein, H.F., & Hill, R.F. (1979). Adaptive modalities among Slovak- and Polish-Americans: Some issues in cultural continuity and change. *Anthropology, 3*(1-2), 95-107.

Stein, H.F. Stanhope, W.D., & Hill, R.F. (1981). P.A. and M.D.—Some parallels with clinical psychology and psychiatry. *Social Science and Medicine, 15E,* 83-93.

Stierlin, H. (1976). *Adolf Hitler: A family perspective.* New York: The Psychohistory Press.

Stoller, R.J. (1975). *Perversion.* New York: Pantheon.

Suzan, M. (1973, August-September). *Magyarization of Hungarian ethnography (1889-1919).* Paper presented at the Ninth International Congress of Anthropological and Ethnological Sciences, Chicago, IL

Thomas, A., Birch, E.G., Chess, S., Hertzig, M.E., & Korn, S. (1963), *Behavioral individuality in early childhood.* New York: University Press.

Turner, V. (1977). Process, system, and symbol: A new anthropological synthesis. *Daedalus, 10*(3), 61-80.

van der Waals, H.G. (1952). Discussion of the mutual influences in the development of ego and id. *The psychoanalytic study of the child, 7,* 66-68.

Volkan, V.D. (1972). The birds of Cyprus: A psychopolitical observation. *American Journal of Psychotherapy, 26,* 378-383.

Volkan, V.D. (1979). *Cyprus—War and adaptation.* Charlottesville, VA: University Press of Virginia.

Volkan, V.D. (1980). Narcissistic personality organization and reparative leadership. *International Journal of Group Psychotherapy, 30,* 131-152.

Volkan, V.D. (1981). *Linking objects and linking phenomena.* New York: International Universities Press.

Volkan, V.D. (1985). The need to have enemies and allies: A developmental approach. *Political Psychology, 6,* 219-247.

Volkan, V.D. (1986). "Suitable targets of externalization" and schizophrenia. In D.B. Feinsilver (Ed.), *Toward a comprehensive model for schizophrenic disorders* (pp. 125-153). New York: Analytic Press.

Volkan, V.D., & Itzkowitz, N. (1984). *The immortal Ataturk*. Chicago: University of Chicago Press.

Wallace, A.F.C. (1956). Revitalization movements. *American Anthropologist, 58,* 264-281.

Walsh, M.N., & Scandalis, B.G. (1975). Male initiation rites and modern warfare as related expressions of unconscious cross-generational aggression. In M.A. Nettleship, R.D. Givens, & A. Nettleship (Eds.), *War: Its causes and correlates.* The Hague: Mouton.

Weber, M. (1967). *The theory of social and economic organization* (A.M. Henderson & T. Parsons, Trans.) New York: Oxford University Press.

Webster's New Collegiate Dictionary (1977), Springfield, PA: G. & C. Merriam Co.

Westlundh, B., & Smith, G. (1983). Perceptgenesis and the psychodynamics of perception. *Psychoanalysis and Contemporary Thought, 6*(4), 597-640.

Wilson, E.O. (1975). *Sociobiology: The new synthesis.* Cambridge: Belknap Press (Harvard).

Winnicott, D.W. (1953). Transitional objects and transitional phenomena. *International Journal of Psycho-Analysis, 34,* 89-97.

Winnicott, D.W. (1965). *The maturational processes and the facilitating environment: Studies in the theory of emotional development.* New York: International Universities Press.

Wolfenstein, M. (1966). How is mourning possible? *The psychoanalytic study of the child, 21,* 93-123.

Wynne, L.C. (1965). Some indications and contraindications for exploratory family therapy. In I. Boszormenyi-Nagy & J.L. Framo (Eds.), *Intensive family therapy: Theoretical and practical aspects* (pp. 289-322). New York: Harper & Row. (Reprinted 1985, New York: Brunner/Mazel)

Yeats, W.B. (1959, fifth printing) *The collected poems of W.B. Yeats* (p. 249). New York: The Macmillan Company.

Yu, K.H., & Kim, L.I.C. (1983), The growth and development of Korean-American children. In G.J. Powell, J. Yamamoto, A. Romero, & A. Morales (Eds.), *The psychosocial development of minority group children* (pp. 147-166). New York: Brunner/Mazel.

Zenner, W.P. (1970). Jokes and ethnic stereotyping. *Anthropological Quarterly, 43,* 93-113.

INDEX

GAP COMMITTEES AND MEMBERSHIP

COMMITTEE ON ADOLESCENCE
Clarice J. Kestenbaum, New York, N.Y.,
 Chairperson
Hector R. Bird, New York, N.Y.
Ian A. Canino, New York, N.Y.
Warren J. Gadpaille, Denver, Colo.
Michael G. Kalogerakis, New York,
 N.Y.
Silvio J. Onesti, Jr., Belmont, Mass.

COMMITTEE ON AGING
Gene D. Cohen, Washington, D.C.,
 Chairperson
Eric D. Caine, Rochester, N.Y.
Charles M. Gaitz, Houston, Tex.
Gabe J. Maletta, Minneapolis, Minn.
Robert J. Nathan, Philadelphia, Pa.
George H. Pollock, Chicago, Ill.
Kenneth M. Sakauye, Chicago, Ill.
Charles A. Shamoian, Larchmont, N.Y.
F. Conyers Thompson, Jr., Atlanta, Ga.

COMMITTEE ON ALCOHOLISM AND THE
 ADDICTIONS
Edward J. Khantzian, Haverhill, Mass.,
 Chairperson
Richard J. Frances, Newark, N.J.
Sheldon I. Miller, Newark, N.J.
Robert B. Millman, New York, N.Y.
Steven M. Mirin, Westwood, Mass.
Edgar P. Nace, Dallas, Tex.
Norman L. Paul, Lexington, Mass.
Bruce J. Rounsaville, Woodbridge,
 Conn.

COMMITTEE ON CHILD PSYCHIATRY
Theodore Shapiro, New York, N.Y.,
 Chairperson
James M. Bell, Canaan, N.Y.
Harlow Donald Dunton, New York, N.Y.
Joseph Fischhoff, Detroit, Mich.
John F. McDermott, Jr., Honolulu,
 Hawaii
John Schowalter, New Haven, Conn.
Peter E. Tanguay, Los Angeles, Calif.
Lenore Terr, San Francisco, Calif.

COMMITTEE ON COLLEGE STUDENTS
Myron B. Liptzin, Chapel Hill, N.C.,
 Chairperson
Robert L. Arnstein, Hamden, Conn.
Varda Backus, La Jolla, Calif.
Harrison P. Eddy, New York, N.Y.
Malkah Tolpin Notman, Brookline,
 Mass.
Gloria C. Onque, Pittsburgh, Pa.
Elizabeth Aub Reid, Cambridge, Mass.
Earle Silber, Chevy Chase, Md.
Tom G. Stauffer, White Plains, N.Y.

COMMITTEE ON CULTURAL PSYCHIATRY
Ezra E.H. Griffith, New Haven, Conn.,
 Chairperson
Edward F. Foulks, New Orleans, La.
Pedro Ruiz, Houston, Tex.
John P. Spiegel, Waltham, Mass.
Ronald M. Wintrob, Providence, R.I.
Joe Yamamoto, Los Angeles, Calif.

William H. Hetznecker, Philadelphia,
Pa.
Harris B. Peck, New Rochelle, N.Y.
Naomi Rae-Grant, London, Ontario
Morton M. Silverman, Bethesda, Md.
Anne Marie Wolf-Schatz,
Conshohocken, Pa.

COMMITTEE ON PSYCHIATRY AND THE
COMMUNITY
Kenneth Minkoff, Woburn, Mass.,
Chairperson
C. Knight Aldrich, Charlottesville, Va.
David G. Greenfield, Guilford, Conn.
H. Richard Lamb, Los Angeles, Calif.
John C. Nemiah, Hanover, N.H.
Rebecca L. Potter, Tucson, Ariz.
Alexander S. Rogawski, Los Angeles,
Calif.
John J. Schwab, Louisville, Ky.
John A. Talbott, Baltimore, Md.
Charles B. Wilkinson, Kansas City, Mo.

COMMITTEE ON PSYCHIATRY AND LAW
Jonas R. Rappeport, Baltimore, Md.,
Chairperson
Park E. Dietz, Charlottesville, Va.
John Donnelly, Hartford, Conn.
Carl P. Malmquist, Minneapolis, Minn.
Herbert C. Modlin, Topeka, Kans.
Phillip J. Resnick, Cleveland, Ohio
Loren H. Roth, Pittsburgh, Pa.
Joseph Satten, San Francisco, Calif.
William D. Weitzel, Lexington, Ky.
Howard V. Zonana, New Haven, Conn.

COMMITTEE ON PSYCHIATRY AND
RELIGION
Albert J. Lubin, Woodside, Calif.,
Chairperson
Sidney Furst, Bronx, N.Y.
Richard C. Lewis, New Haven, Conn.
Earl A. Loomis, Jr., Augusta, Ga.

Abigail R. Ostow, Belmont, Mass.
Mortimer Ostow, Bronx, N.Y.
Sally K. Severino, White Plains, N.Y.
Clyde R. Snyder, Fayetteville, N.C.

COMMITTEE ON PSYCHIATRY IN INDUSTRY
Barrie S. Greiff, Newton, Mass.,
Chairperson
Peter L. Brill, Philadelphia, Pa.
Duane Q. Hagen, St. Louis, Mo.
R. Edward Huffman, Asheville, N.C.
David E. Morrison, Palatine, Ill.
David B. Robbins, Chappaqua, N.Y.
Jay B. Rohrlich, New York, N.Y.
Clarence J. Rowe, St. Paul, Minn.
Jeffrey L. Speller, Alexandria, Va.

COMMITTEE ON PSYCHOPATHOLOGY
David A. Adler, Boston, Mass.,
Chairperson
Jeffrey Berlant, Summit, N.J.
Robert E. Drake, Hanover, N.H.
James M. Ellison, Watertown, Mass.
Howard H. Goldman, Rockville, Md.
Richard E. Renneker, Los Angeles,
Calif.

COMMITTEE ON PUBLIC EDUCATION
Keith H. Johansen, Dallas, Tex.,
Chairperson
Susan J. Blumenthal, Washington, D.C.
Steven E. Katz, New York, N.Y.
Robert A. Solow, Beverly Hills, Calif.
Kenneth N. Vogtsberger, San Antonio,
Tex.

COMMITTEE ON RESEARCH
Robert Cancro, New York, N.Y.,
Chairperson
Kenneth Z. Altshuler, Dallas, Tex.
Jack A. Grebb, New York, N.Y.
John H. Greist, Madison, Wisc.

Jerry M. Lewis, Dallas, Tex.
Morris A. Lipton, Chapel Hill,
N.C.
John G. Looney, Durham, N.C.
Sidney Malitz, New York, N.Y.
Zebulon Taintor, Orangeburg, N.Y.

COMMITTEE ON SOCIAL ISSUES
Ian E. Alger, New York, N.Y.,
Chairperson
William R. Beardslee, Boston, Mass.
Judith H. Gold, Halifax, Nova
Scotia
Roderic Gorney, Los Angeles, Calif.
Martha J. Kirkpatrick, Los Angeles,
Calif.
Perry Ottenberg, Philadelphia, Pa.
Kendon W. Smith, Piermont, N.Y.

COMMITTEE ON THERAPEUTIC CARE
Milton Kramer, Cincinnati, Ohio,
Chairperson
Bernard Bandler, Cambridge, Mass.
Thomas E. Curtis, Chapel Hill, N.C.
Donald W. Hammersley, Washington,
D.C.
William B. Hunter, III, Albuquerque,
N.M.
Roberto L. Jimenez, San Antonio, Tex.
William W. Richards, Anchorage,
Aka.

COMMITTEE ON THERAPY
Allen D. Rosenblatt, La Jolla, Calif.,
Chairperson
Jules R. Bemporad, Boston, Mass.
Henry W. Brosin, Tucson, Ariz.
Eugene B. Feigelson, Brooklyn, N.Y.
Robert Michels, New York, N.Y.
Andrew P. Morrison, Cambridge,
Mass.
William C. Offenkrantz, Milwaukee,
Wis.

CONTRIBUTING MEMBERS
John E. Adams, Gainesville, Fl.
Carlos C. Alden, Jr., Buffalo, N.Y.

Spencer Bayles, Houston, Tex.
C. Christian Beels, New York, N.Y.
Elissa P. Benedek, Ann Arbor, Mich.
Sidney Berman, Washington, D.C.
H. Keith H. Brodie, Durham, N.C.
Charles M. Bryant, San Francisco,
Calif.
Ewald W. Busse, Durham, N.C.
Robert N. Butler, New York, N.Y.

Eugene M. Caffey, Jr., Bowie, Md.
Ian L.W. Clancey, Ontario, Canada
Sanford I. Cohen, Boston, Mass.

James S. Eaton, Jr., Washington, D.C.
Lloyd C. Elam, Nashville, Tenn.
Stanley H. Eldred, Belmont, Mass.
Joseph T. English, New York, N.Y.
Louis C. English, Pomona, N.Y.

Sherman C. Feinstein, Highland Park,
Ill.
Archie R. Foley, New York, N.Y.
Daniel X. Freedman, Los Angeles,
Calif.

Henry J. Gault, Highland Park, Ill.
Alexander Gralnick, Port Chester, N.Y.
Joseph M. Green, Madison, Wis.
Milton Greenblatt, Sylmar, Calif.
Lawrence F. Greenleigh, Los Angeles,
Calif.
Jon E. Gudeman, Milwaukee, Wisc.

Seymour L. Halleck, Chapel Hill,
N.C.
Stanley Hammons, Lexington, Ky.
J. Cotter Hirschberg, Topeka, Kans.

Jay Katz, New Haven, Conn.
James A. Knight, New Orleans, La.
Othilda M. Krug, Cincinnati, Ohio

Alan I. Levenson, Tucson, Ariz.
Ruth W. Lidz, Woodbridge, Conn.
Orlando B. Lightfoot, Boston, Mass.
Reginald S. Lourie, Chevy Chase, Md.
Norman L. Loux, Sellersville, Pa.

John A. MacLeod, Cincinnati, Ohio
Leo Madow, Philadelphia, Pa.
Charles A. Malone, Cleveland, Ohio
Peter A. Martin, Lake Orion, Mich.
Ake Mattsson, Danderyd, Sweden
Alan A. McLean, Westport, Conn.
David Mendell, Houston, Tex.
Roy W. Menninger, Topeka, Kans.
Mary E. Mercer, Nyack, N.Y.
Derek Miller, Chicago, Ill.
Richard D. Morrill, Boston, Mass.

Joseph D. Noshpitz, Washington, D.C.

Bernard L. Pacella, New York, N.Y.
Herbert Pardes, New York, N.Y.
Marvin E. Perkins, Salem, Va.

David N. Ratnavale, Bethesda, Md.
Kent E. Robinson, Towson, Md.
W. Donald Ross, Cincinnati, Ohio
Lester H. Rudy, Chicago, Ill.
George E. Ruff, Philadelphia, Pa.

David S. Sanders, Los Angeles, Calif.
Donald J. Scherl, Brooklyn, N.Y.
Charles Shagrass, Philadelphia, Pa.
Miles F. Shore, Boston, Mass.
Albert J. Silverman, Ann Arbor, Mich.
Benson R. Snyder, Cambridge, Mass.
David A. Soskis, Bala Cynwyd, Pa.
Jeanne Spurlock, Washington, D.C.
Brandt F. Steele, Denver, Colo.
Alan A. Stone, Cambridge, Mass.
Robert E. Switzer, Dunn Loring, Va.

Perry C. Talkington, Dallas, Tex.
Bryce Templeton, Philadelphia, Pa.
Prescott W. Thompson, Beaverton,
Oreg.

Joe P. Tupin, Sacramento, Calif.
John A. Turner, San Francisco, Calif.

Gene L. Usdin, New Orleans, La.

Warren T. Vaughan, Jr., Portola Valley,
Calif.

Andrew S. Watson, Ann Arbor, Mich.
Joseph B. Wheelwright, Kentfield,
Calif.
Robert L. Williams, Houston, Tex.
Paul Tyler Wilson, Bethesda, Md.
Sherwyn M. Woods, Los Angeles,
Calif.

Kent A. Zimmerman, Berkeley, Calif.
Israel Zwerling, Philadelphia, Pa.

LIFE MEMBERS
C. Knight Aldrich, Charlottesville, Va.
Bernard Bandler, Cambridge, Mass.
Walter E. Barton, Hartland, Vt.
Viola W. Bernard, New York, N.Y.
Wilfred Bloomberg, Cambridge, Mass.
Murray Bowen, Chevy Chase, Md.
Henry W. Brosin, Tucson, Ariz.
John Donnelly, Hartford, Conn.
Merrill T. Eaton, Omaha, Neb.
O. Spurgeon English, Narberth, Pa.
Stephen Fleck, New Haven, Conn.
Jerome Frank, Baltimore, Md.
Robert S. Garber, Osprey, Fl.
Robert I. Gibson, Towson, Md.
Paul E. Huston, Iowa City, Iowa
Margaret M. Lawrence, Pomona, N.Y.
Harold I. Lief, Philadelphia, Pa.
Morris A. Lipton, Chapel Hill, N.C.
Judd Marmor, Los Angeles, Calif.
Karl A. Menninger, Topeka, Kans.
Herbert C. Modlin, Topeka, Kans.
John C. Nemiah, Hanover, N.H.
Mabel Ross, Sun City, Ariz.
Julius Schreiber, Washington, D.C.
George Tarjan, Los Angeles, Calif.

Jack A. Wolford, Pittsburgh, Pa.
Henry H. Work, Bethesda, Md.

BOARD OF DIRECTORS

OFFICERS

President
Jerry M. Lewis
Timberlawn Foundation
P.O. Box 270789
Dallas, Tex. 75227

President-Elect
Carolyn B. Robinowitz
Deputy Medical Director
American Psychiatric Association
1400 K Street, N.W.
Washington, D.C. 20005

Secretary
Allan Beigel
30 Camino Español
Tucson, Ariz. 85716

Treasurer
Charles B. Wilkinson
600 E. 22nd Street
Kansas City, Mo. 64108

Board Members
David R. Hawkins
Silvio J. Onesti
John A. Talbott
Lenore Terr

Past Presidents
*William C. Menninger	1946–51
Jack R. Ewalt	1951–53
Walter E. Barton	1953–55
*Sol W. Ginsburg	1955–57
*Dana L. Farnsworth	1957–59
*Marion E. Kenworthy	1959–61
Henry W. Brosin	1961–63
*Leo H. Bartemeier	1963–65

Robert S. Garber	1965–67
Herbert C. Modlin	1967–69
John Donnelly	1969–71
George Tarjan	1971–73
Judd Marmor	1973–75
John C. Nemiah	1975–77
Jack A. Wolford	1977–79
Robert W. Gibson	1979–81
*Jack Weinberg	1981–82
Henry H. Work	1982–85
Michael R. Zales	1985–87

PUBLICATIONS BOARD

Chairman
Alexander S. Rogawski
11665 W. Olympic Blvd. #302
Los Angeles, CA 90064

C. Knight Aldrich
Robert L. Arnstein
Milton Kramer
W. Walter Menninger
Robert A. Solow

Consultant
John C. Nemiah

Ex-Officio
Jerry M. Lewis
Carolyn B. Robinowitz

CONTRIBUTORS
Abbott Laboratories
American Charitable Fund
Dr. and Mrs. Richard Aron
Mr. Robert C. Baker
Maurice Falk Medical Fund
Mrs. Carol Gold
Grove Foundation, Inc.
Miss Gayle Groves

---

*deceased

Ittleson Foundation, Inc.
Mr. Barry Jacobson
Mrs. Allan H. Kalmus
Marion E. Kenworthy—Sarah H.
  Swift Foundation, Inc.
Mr. Larry Korman
McNeil Pharmaceutical
Phillips Foundation

Sandoz, Inc.
Smith Kline Beckman Corporation
Tappanz Foundation, Inc.
The Upjohn Company
van Amerigen Foundation, Inc.
Wyeth Laboratories
Mr. and Mrs. William A. Zales

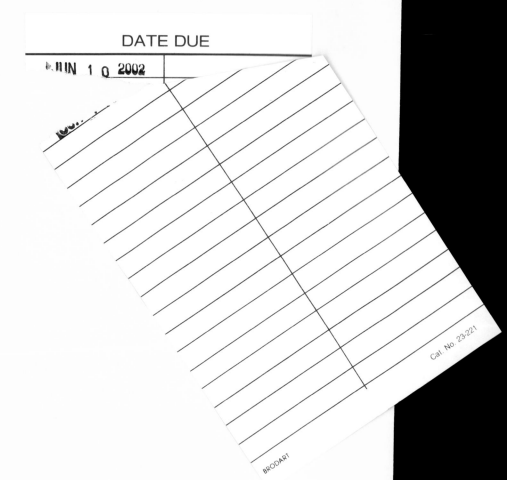